Cruel Lives

For my mother, Alice
Born Hunslet, August 1913
Died Cleckheaton, January 2011.

She witnessed many of the diseases listed here,
but lived to see great improvements in housing and health.

Cruel Lives

A History of Some West Yorkshire Epidemics

John Brooke

Rastrick High School

© 2012 John Brooke

Published by Rastrick High School
Field Top Road
Rastrick
Brighouse
HD6 3XB
Email: cruellives@btinternet.com

All rights reserved. No part of this publication may be reproduced,
stored in a retrieval system, or transmitted in any form
or by any means, electronic, mechanical, photocopying, recording or otherwise,
without the prior permission of the publishers.

ISBN: 978-0-9545391-1-5

Typeset in Garamond
Page layout by Highlight Type Bureau Ltd
Bradford BD8 7HB
Printed and bound in Great Britain by
The Amadeus Press, West 26 Business Park
Cleckheaton, BD19 4TQ

The proceeds from the sale of this book will be donated to
Overgate Hospice, Elland, HX5 0QY

Contents

Foreword vi
Preface vii
1 Introductory Chapter. The Epidemic Streets: Housing and Health in Victorian Britain 1
2 The Fatal Effects of a Malady: Measles in Leeds in 1809 and 1891 12
3 A Tidal Wave of Disease: The 1832 Leeds Cholera Epidemic 22
4 An Aggravated Calamity: Heptonstall-Slack 1843-44. Typhus or Typhoid? .. 44
5 A Farmer, a Hired Man and a Milk Round:
  The 1880-81 Halifax Scarlet Fever Epidemic 53
6 A Memorable Visitation: The 1881 Spen Valley Influenza Epidemic 70
7 When Panic Seized the Town: The Brighouse Smallpox Epidemic 83
8 A Baffling Outbreak: Diphtheria in Bradford, 1906 111
9 An Unwelcome Present from Scarborough:
  The 1932 Denby Dale Typhoid Outbreak 123

List of Figures 149
List of Tables 151
Notes 152
Index 170
List of Subscribers 179

Foreword by Professor Geoff Gill, BA, MA, PhD, MD, FRCP, DTM&H

In this fascinating book, we are given an insight into the desperately serious problem of infectious disease in Britain in the nineteenth and early twentieth centuries. John Brooke takes us through epidemics in west Yorkshire between 1809 and 1932, involving such diseases as measles, influenza, cholera, smallpox, typhoid, typhus, diphtheria and scarlet fever. All of these are meticulously researched and academically presented, but are intriguing and immensely readable tales. These stories are also by no means only of relevance to the locality of Yorkshire; the book is a good example of what social historians call 'micro to macro' or 'from the particular to the general'. What was going on in this particular part of the north of England was very typical of the situation elsewhere in Britain.

A number of the diseases described in this book are now confined to tropical countries – cholera, typhoid and typhus for example. This demonstrates that such diseases do not necessarily need a warm climate to flourish, but require only a susceptible human population and the ability of the infecting organism to flourish both outside and inside the host. The nineteenth century was certainly a time when such conditions existed in Britain. The population was rapidly expanding and the industrial revolution led to massive rural-urban migration. Sanitation and fresh water supply did not exist in the early nineteenth century, and was not universal until the later parts of the nineteenth and early twentieth century. Overcrowding and poor nutrition added to population susceptibility to infective disease, and mortality (particularly in infants and children) was massive. Simply reaching adult life in the 1830s and 1840s was a bonus, and survival to old age was rare.

As well as the 'classic' infectious diseases described in this book, it is worth remembering that simple gastro-enteritis and pneumonia probably accounted for the majority of infective deaths. Poor nutrition also turned mild or moderate infections into life-threatening illnesses, notably measles (which is still a major killer of poorly nourished children in the 3rd World). Also, for much of the times covered in this book, the modes of transmission of these diseases were quite unknown, and no effective treatments existed. Thus, prior to the pioneering work of Dr John Snow in London in 1854, the water-borne transmission of cholera was not appreciated, and it was thought to be spread by bad smells (or miasma) in the air. Treatment involved brandy and opium for the fortunate, and enemas and purgatives for the not-so-lucky!

Of the diseases described in this book, only influenza is still of concern in modern Britain. Antibiotics, immunisation, clean water, effective sanitation and better housing have all contributed to the triumph over these epidemic infections. But history may, of course, be revisited upon us if we do not learn its lessons, and John Brooke's book on 'Cruel Lives' is a useful reminder of these dark and dangerous times in the not so distant past.

Geoff Gill
Professor of International Medicine
Liverpool School of Tropical Medicine

Preface

As the sub-title indicates, this book is a study of some West Yorkshire epidemics. It is not in any way intended to be a complete history of these events. The epidemics chronicled have been chosen to provide a representative selection of the diseases that were prevalent in the nineteenth and early twentieth centuries. The selection from within each category resulted in the choice of an outbreak that was either particularly interesting or unusual. In the case of some diseases the selection was not difficult and I could, for example, have chosen any number of measles epidemics.

The starting point for each of the selections has been wide and varied. The cholera chapter grew out of my previous involvement in a project with the Thackray Medical Museum; the smallpox chapter began initially when I was involved as a visiting history tutor at Rastrick High School some eight years ago, and my friend, Ron Jackson, drew my attention to the Denby Dale typhoid outbreak. I had known about the Spen Valley influenza outbreak for almost fifty years, after researching a Cleckheaton church history in 1964; the story of the farmer and the Halifax scarlet fever outbreak came to my notice through my inclination to follow a lead provided by footnotes in a range of books dealing with public health; the Heptonstall-Slack epidemic was brought to my notice by a number of local historians familiar with the Calder Valley. Finally, I came across the measles and diphtheria epidemics after trawling through many medical officers of health and Local Government Board reports, and burial records.

None of these stories would have been recorded here, though, if it had not been for the generous help and advice received from many people during the course of researching and writing. Some may only have made a brief comment or suggested a lead but I hope that they will accept my general thanks as their ideas have often proved to be invaluable. Others have been more closely involved and deserve special thanks.

The book had its origins in Rastrick High School when I was working with a small group of students on a project recording a smallpox epidemic. I am grateful, therefore, that Mrs. Helen Lennie, the headteacher, was happy to support my idea that the school publish this further work. I shared my initial ideas with Professor Geoffrey Gill, with whom I had worked on the cholera project and he, along with Dr. Steven Chambers and Dr. Alan Greenwood, have not only read sections of the manuscript but offered advice when I was floundering with the more technical aspects of a disease. I am grateful for their knowledge, support and tolerance.

Ron Jackson's technical background has been invaluable throughout my Denby Dale epidemic investigations and he, along with many others, has given much in the way of local knowledge and personal memories. John Springer provided vital information about the Robson family and Quaker Bottom. This enabled me to locate Kitty Robson's ancestors and her grandson, James Anderson, has been exceptionally helpful and understanding. Without his agreement the story would have been so much less poignant. David Cook, a High Flatts farmer helped on many occasions to locate drains in his fields and has been particularly obliging. Mrs. Mary Lockwood and her son Michael, the late Philip Parker and Mrs. Marjorie Parker, Stephen Howes and Barry Natton have willingly let me have information relating to their, in some cases tragic, family links with the outbreak and have been especially helpful. Alex Hollweg was equally helpful when I was researching the Spen Valley influenza epidemic and his family's connections with the outbreak.

The staff at the West Yorkshire Archives in Bradford, Calderdale (Halifax) and Kirklees (Huddersfield), Leeds and Wakefield, along with reference library staff in Halifax, Leeds and Huddersfield never failed to be patient, obliging and knowledgeable. The Wellcome Library and the British Library Newspaper Library in London have proved to be a rich source of material, and staff there have always been willing to offer advice. More locally, I have gained much from my visits to the Health Sciences and Brotherton Libraries in Leeds. Margaret Heward at the Spenborough Guardian office in Cleckheaton has been especially kind. My next door neighbours Nev and Liz Leah have, as in the past, responded willingly to my many requests for assistance. Nev has always been willing to offer advice when I was struggling to make sense of my computer and Liz has researched families, on my behalf, and fleshed out what were, initially, tenuous links with some of the outbreaks. Alan Petford has never refused my requests for help, and his experience and knowledge in relation to a number of local publications has been extremely beneficial. Andrew Tatham provided both help and advice with the index. David Crossland at The Amadeus Press and Angela Lawless at Highlight Type Bureau Ltd have been helpful, tolerant and agreeable.

During the book's final stages, the help of Bob Horne has been invaluable. Not only has he cast an assiduous eye over the whole work and used his red pen both skilfully and tactfully, he has also offered patient and constructive advice throughout. My understanding of when to use the Oxford comma, square brackets, and a hyphen in certain words has improved considerably! I owe him a debt of considerable gratitude. Errors that remain are, of course, my responsibility.

John Brooke
Lightcliffe, Halifax
April 2012.

Chapter One

The Epidemic Streets

Housing and Health in Nineteenth-Century Britain

Introduction

Poverty, overcrowding and inadequate sanitation had a profound effect on the lives of those condemned to a miserable existence in the rapidly growing towns of nineteenth-century Britain. Epidemic disease could break out anywhere, but it was those in the large industrial towns that were hit the hardest. Unpredictable epidemics caused by lethal microbes found a ready welcome in the filthy streets of communities where population growth was unprecedented. It was not until the establishment of local sanitary departments in the mid nineteenth century, led by medical officers of health (MOH), that the connection between disease and living conditions was accepted or understood.

By the end of the nineteenth century, it was clear that the ravages of many of the infectious diseases were being conquered. Smallpox, typhus and cholera had virtually disappeared from mortality records and typhoid and scarlet fever were following. Not everyone benefited from this improvement and infant mortality, for example, was still unacceptably high. The twentieth century did not, however, see the total eradication of dangerous outbreaks. As we shall see, diphtheria struck in Bradford in 1904, and typhoid in Denby Dale in 1932. Even today many parts of the underdeveloped world suffer epidemics that nineteenth-century Britain experienced, and an outbreak of a lethal microbe occasionally occurs in our own midst.

The evidence surrounding many of the epidemics recorded here is often patchy and contradictory. For example, not all the outbreaks occurred where there was abject poverty and overcrowding. Death and disease did, though, find a greater and ready welcome in the homes of the poorest people living in slum dwellings. However, for all who were subjected to desperately inadequate living conditions, or lived in communities where disease found a home, life was unremittingly cruel.

Population Growth in Industrial Britain

When the first census was taken in 1801, only 30 per cent of the British population of approximately 10.5 million lived in towns, and London accounted for 959,000 of these. By 1851 the 30 per cent had risen to 54 per cent and, by the end of the century, to 78 per cent. The increase in the percentage of people moving from country to town was further augmented by the growth in the population as a whole, which had increased to around forty million by the time of Queen Victoria's death.[1] By 1851 the populations of seven English towns had exceeded one hundred thousand. Liverpool had risen to 395,000, Manchester to 338,000 and, in West Yorkshire, Leeds to 172,000 and Bradford to 104,000.[2] Prior to this century of growth, in what became the industrial centres of the country, the biggest places outside London had been Norwich (the second city in the eighteenth century with thirty thousand people), York and Exeter.[3]

The figures here, however, tend to conceal the phenomenally rapid growth of certain places within a remarkably short period of time. Manchester grew by 40.4 per cent in the decade 1811-21, Liverpool by 43.6 per cent between 1821-31 and Leeds by 47.2 per cent in the same period.[4] In the fifty-year period from 1801 Leeds grew by 224 per cent, Huddersfield by 325 per cent and Bradford by an amazing 682 per cent from just thirteen thousand.[5] It wasn't just the industrial towns that grew quickly. The rapidly developing railway network enabled the expanding middle classes to gain easy access to spa towns, and seaside resorts such as Brighton and Scarborough. By the 1851 census, eleven of the resorts mentioned had grown by no less than 214 per cent since 1801.[6]

Table 1:1 Population growth, in thousands, amongst major West Yorkshire towns: 1801-1851 [7]

	1801	1811	1821	1831	1841	1851
Bradford	13	16	26	44	67	104
Halifax	12	13	17	22	28	34
Huddersfield	7	10	13	19	25	31
Leeds	53	63	84	123	152	172
Wakefield	11	11	14	16	19	22

According to John Burnett, the processes of town growth were both local and individual and do not appear, in his view, to fit into any pattern. The Health of Towns Committee, established in 1844 did, however, use a simple classification system to identify the variety of English urban development. They listed the metropolis, manufacturing towns, seaport towns, great watering places and 'county and inland towns, not the seat of any particular manufacture'. English towns in general were not planned. They grew by expansion outwards and by infilling within existing boundaries. Nearness to places of work was the main reason for clustering and overcrowding.[8] Centres of cities that were once home to the wealthier residents, the commercial and professional classes, soon became the poorest quarters as the former occupants departed to the suburbs. This mainly took place post 1850 with the development of what Burnett calls the 'iron-ways', for example the electric tramcar and the rail system both over and underground, although in 1855 it was estimated that twenty thousand people were commuting into London by horse bus.[9]

Despite this increase in travel opportunities, overcrowding, as we shall see, became

The Epidemic Streets

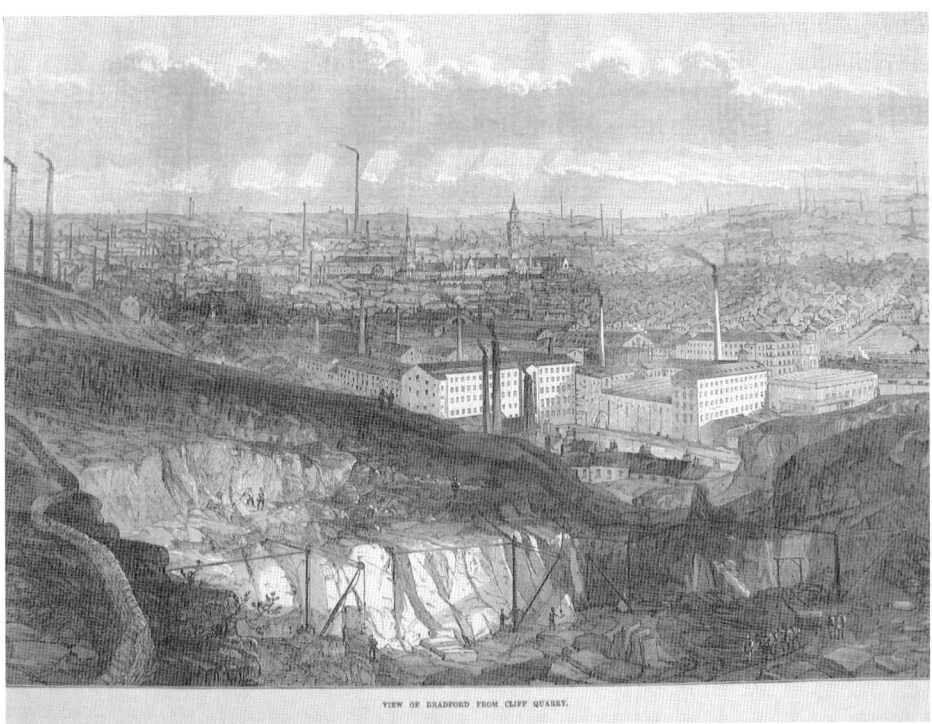

Figure 1:1 *Bradford from Cliff Quarry* 1873.
Illustrated London News: 20 September 1873. *(Yorkshire Archaeological Society)*

commonplace and rogue landlords took advantage of the opportunity presented by the rapid population growth. The Boot and Shoe Yard in Leeds, about which we shall learn much more later, with dwellings that were 'abominably filthy, stinking and destitute'[10] was home to 340 people in thirty-four houses. This was just one example and was said to pay the best annual interest of any property in the borough.[11] The difficulty in remedying this state of things, confirmed James Hole in 1866, was the fact that the 'wretched homes' were indeed highly remunerative to landlords.[12]

There were also other opportunities for planning where a new industry arose in what had often been a sparsely populated area. This applied especially to areas that saw the establishment of a new factory, textile mill, coal pit or railway junction and workshop.The construction of railway towns such as Crewe and Swindon enabled a more planned development to take place. Other well known examples of planned development are the company town or village - the 'model village' - that had its origins well before the nineteenth century with Richard Arkwright at Cromford in 1771, Jedediah Strutt at Belper in 1776 and Samuel Greg at Styal in 1784. Perhaps the best-known development during this time was that at New Lanark, in Scotland. Planning began in 1792 through David Dale, the father-in-law- of Robert Owen who became the second owner in 1813.

The initial developments were followed, often because the builders were dissatisfied with the living conditions of their workers, by those built in the nineteenth century by Edward Akroyd at Copley and later at Akroyden, Halifax; Titus Salt at Saltaire, William Hesketh Lever at Port Sunlight, and the Cadbury brothers, George and Richard, at Bournville. Walter Creese referred to Akroyd, Francis Crossley and Salt as the 'Bradford-Halifax School' of village makers and he said that 'they explored the middle ground of complete dictation and the reversion to a non-industrialised and non-urbanised existence'.[13] Their altruism, says Enid Gouldie, ought not to be discounted. Their wish to improve the lot of their workpeople was quite genuine.[14] These developments were however, as we shall see, the exception and the lives of many workers in industrial towns in the nineteenth century were often surrounded by poverty, overcrowding, inadequate sanitation and early death.

Health and Life Expectancy

The move to the town for those seeking work, and the subsequent increased urbanisation did not result, as indicated, in improved living conditions for the new residents or an improvement in their health. For about forty years from around 1780, death rates had been falling but this trend began to alter from around 1816. Annual death rates were up at 22.4 per thousand in 1838, although in some towns the rate was much higher. In Bradford, for example, the figure was 26.5 in 1851. Overall they remained above twenty until the 1880s, falling to fifteen in the first decade of the twentieth century.[15] Although the overall death rate had, then, improved as the nineteenth century ended, the infant death rate, that is infant mortality within a year of birth, remained constant at around 153 per thousand births[16] and was actually higher at the end of Victoria's reign than at the beginning. Most large industrial towns had figures in excess of 153, (167 was the average in the twenty-eight largest towns) and 220 was a typical figure in Birmingham, Blackburn, Leicester, Liverpool, London, Manchester, Salford and Preston. For every thousand children born, only 780 would be alive within twelve months. John Simon (1816-1904), Medical Officer to the City of London, memorably referred to these areas as 'Herodian Districts'.[17] The figure is now, in 2012, around 4.4 per thousand births.

Forty per cent of the total recorded deaths in, for example, Middlesborough in the years 1871-73 were of children under the age of one year, and deaths of those aged between one and five accounted for a further twenty per cent.[18] In the 'lowest' districts of Manchester Edwin Chadwick, to whom we shall return later, in his seminal report of 1842, *The Sanitary Condition of the Labouring Population of Great Britain*, indicates that of every thousand births, more than 570 will have died before their fifth birthday. Similar figures for Leeds are recorded.[19] Although the civil registration of births and deaths in England and Wales commenced in 1837, it was not until 1874 that they were made compulsory. William Farr estimated that forty thousand still-births went unrecorded every year in England and Wales.[20]

These infants were not just victims of the many diseases prevalent at the time, but also of childbirth practices and the health of the mother. Thousands of babies were born annually to mothers who were underweight and undernourished. Victorian working class diet, for example, often led to rickets which could cause contracted pelvises, making childbirth difficult. The mother's health was also at risk and in his early years at the Registrar-General's office, established in 1837, William Farr recorded the deaths of three thousand mothers every year and in the final years of Victoria's reign 4,400 mothers died in childbirth. The key cause was often puerperal fever, a streptococcal infection of the uterus immediately after birth. This continued, through inadequate use of antiseptics, to the end of the nineteenth century despite the work of Pasteur, Lister and Koch. As Wohl argues, a single factor taken in isolation may not be highly significant, as with many other aspects of health. This changed, however, when poor nutrition was added to other aspects of working class lives, such as damp, cold and overcrowded dwellings and inadequate sanitation.[21]

Life expectancy figures were obviously affected by the high infant mortality rates but other factors played an important part in the chances of survival of all ages. The startling differences in life expectancy during the nineteenth century amongst the different social groups and, even more noticeably, between the rural and industrial areas in England and Wales makes grim reading. These differences are clearly shown below in table 1:2 drawn from Chadwick's 1842 report. The figures also include direct family members.[22]

Table 1:2   Average age of death 1842

	Manchester	Rutlandshire
Professional persons and gentry	38	52
Tradesmen, farmers, shopkeepers	20	41
Mechanics, labourers	17	38

The data for Leeds in 1842 shows that gentlemen and their families (including the professions) lived on average to the age of forty-five; tradesmen and their families to twenty-six and labourers, servants and mechanics to sixteen.[23] Burnett compares overall figures in England and Wales in 1841, when life expectancy was 41, with the figures for Liverpool (26) and Manchester (24). He adds that similar differences, though not as dramatic, could be shown between healthy and unhealthy districts in the same town.[24] Lampard notes that 'a Manchester born man in Manchester might expect to live just over half as long as his country cousin'.[25] As late in the century as 1893 these variations were still noticeable.[26] In selected 'healthy districts' the life expectancy was 51.48 and in Manchester 27.78. It wasn't just the larger towns that suffered from poor living conditions and lack of adequate sanitation. In Haworth in 1850, 41.6 per-cent of people died before the age of six and the average age of all deaths there was 25.8 years.[27] One of the key factors linked to most of the above was the often inadequate housing provision that a vast majority of the population of towns had to endure.

Housing: Poor quality, overcrowding, inadequate sanitation

The housing provision in towns had caused concern to many with enlightened minds for some time. As early as 1840 Robert Cowan in Scotland had indicated that 'the rapid increase in the amount of the labouring population without any corresponding amount of accommodation being provided for them has been the chief causes of the great mortality in the city of Glasgow'[28] His comments were an early recognition, two years before Chadwick reported, that poor housing, defective sanitation and deficient nutrition led to waste of life through disease, debility and death.[29] The health situation in the Victorian City was seen as a 'consequence of its evolution'.[30] Overcrowding was rife and was really not recognised by politicians and the public to be the most critical aspect of the slum problem until the 1880s.[31] This was in spite of those with enlightened minds identifying the problem thirty years earlier. For example, in 1856 the Medical Officer for the Strand noted that 'overcrowding and disease mutually act and react upon each other'.[32]

He was not alone in his views. Around the same time the MOH for Finsbury, George Newton, was noting the link between overcrowding and high rates of phthisis (consumption) and zymotic (infectious) diseases.[33] Even earlier in Victoria's reign Thomas Southwood Smith had shown that living conditions were the greatest threats to life in the industrial communities. His granddaughter, Octavia Hill, continued much of his work related to housing and health.[34] The problem was not, however, easily addressed as one Dr. Tripe, MOH for Hackney, noted that had he carried out the overcrowding clause in the 1866 Sanitary Act, ten thousand people would have had to sleep on the streets.[35] Industrialisation had, then, a profound effect on the nature of towns, and people's health. When referring to poor housing, inadequate sanitation and lack of space. James Hole wrote in 1866 that:

The inhabitant whose memory can carry him back thirty years recalls pictures of rural beauty, suburban mansions and farmsteads, green fields, waving trees and clear streams where fish could live - where now can be seen only streets, factories and workshops and a river as black as ink.[36]

Others had a similar story to tell. Frederick Engels devotes page after page in the *Conditions of the Working Class in England* to housing, sanitation and street cleansing. In London he came across houses that were 'occupied from cellar to garret, filthy within and without, and their appearance is such that no human being could possibly live in them'.[37] In Bradford the whole town on weekdays was enveloped in a grey cloud of coal smoke, and in Huddersfield he noted that 'filth of every sort lies accumulating, festers and rots, in consequence the adjoining buildings must inevitably be bad and filthy so that in such places diseases arise and threaten the health of the whole town'.[38]

In September, 1865 Clifford Allbutt, physician to the Leeds House of Recovery wrote the following letter to the Leeds Mercury to express his concerns about the housing and general living conditions of so many:

This is no description of a plague stricken town in the fifteenth-century; it is, in faint effort to describe the squalor, the deadliness and the decay of a mass of huts which lies in the town of Leeds between York Street and Marsh Lane; a place of darkness and cruel habitations, within a stone's throw of the Parish Church, where fever is bred…Riley's Yard* is horribly filthy. Look into any others and *see places that fill the fever hospital and he [a visitor] will gain his knowledge at the price of a nausea and an oppression at the epigastrium which will not leave him for hours.*[39]

In Leeds, the River Aire was virtually the town sewer and full of an array of deadly ingredients. It was described in 1840 as being:

Full of refuse from water closets, cesspools, privies, common drains, dung hill drainings, infirmary refuse, waste from slaughter houses, chemical soap, pig manure, blue and black dye, dead animals, vegetable substances and occasionally a decomposed human body.[40]

It wasn't just the housing and the state of the streets that was giving those with enlightened minds cause for concern. John Ruskin turned his attention to the mills and the poisoned atmosphere for which they were responsible. The workers were at risk from the dangers within and he recorded that the fine clothes produced under conditions 'so destructive to human life and happiness that those who wear them have entered into partnership with death, and dressed themselves in his spoils'.[41]

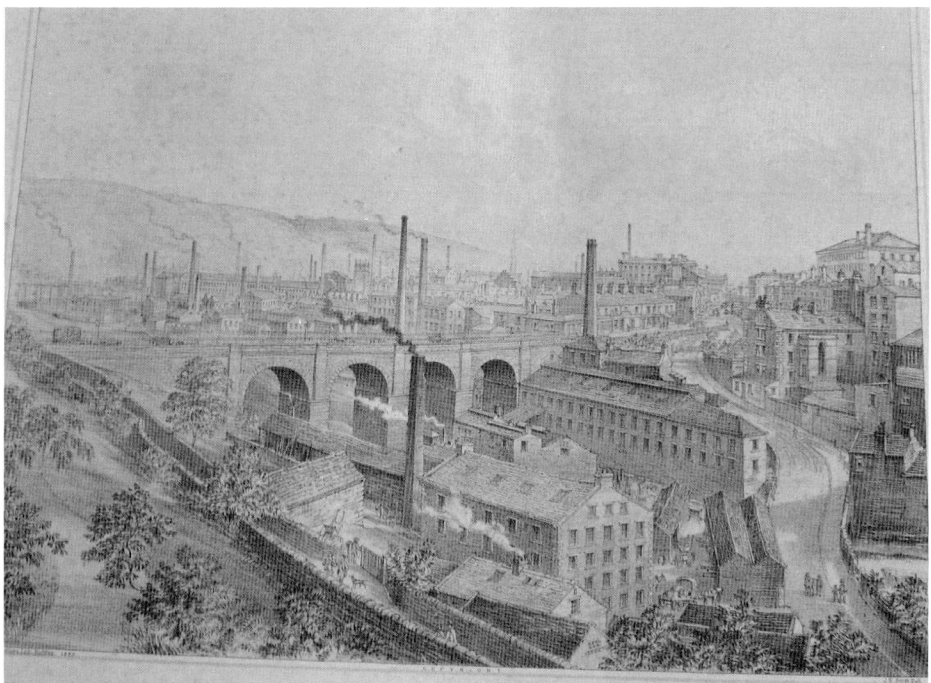

Figure 1:2 Halifax: North Bridge and Bowling Dyke, 1864
(*Yorkshire Archaeological Society*)

This view from the Mount, Haley Hill by Joseph Rideal Smith (1837-1915) shows the stone bridge that was demolished in 1870 to be replaced by the present construction.[42]

---

*Riley's Yard was noted by Robert Baker (see chapter three) in his report to the Leeds Board of Health in 1833, as a cause for concern. It was, he reported, confined and dirty, with many inhabitants.[43]

The appalling state of the housing provision for the working people of England and Wales also featured in many nineteenth-century works of fiction. Elizabeth Gaskell gives us a vivid picture of the Davenports' home in *Mary Barton,* a world that was far removed from *Cranford.* The street where their home was located was unpaved and down the middle ran a gutter into which 'women tossed household slops of every description. The cellar was very dark indeed and the smell was so foetid and almost knocked down those entering'. Children were rolling in the wet damp floor into which the stagnant filthy moisture of the street oozed up.[44] Charles Dickens wrote in *Little Dorrit* that in London, through the heart of the town, a deadly sewer ebbed and flowed, in place of the fine fresh river.[45] In *Hard Times* the fictional Coketown, (an amalgam of Preston, Oldham and Manchester)[46], there was a black canal and a river that 'ran purple with ill smelling dye'.[47] William Ranger noted, in his 1851 report on Halifax, that the close pent-up air in the dwellings of the poorer classes deteriorates their health and 'degenerates their bodily functions'.[48]

These then were the conditions in which the people, Chadwick's 'Labouring Population of Great Britain',[49] made their homes with unerring frequency, and died from both epidemic and endemic diseases. Chadwick's report was one of the seminal works of nineteenth-century social history and ran to over 400 pages of reports, case studies and the author's carefully argued opinions. Halliday indicates that the report is chiefly concerned with four themes. The key element was Chadwick's identification of the relationship between living conditions and disease. This will prove to be a recurring theme as we consider a range of epidemics. His other concerns were the need for new systems of administration; the social effects, such as intemperance and immorality, of poor living conditions; the cost of disease arising from the creation of widows and those rendered incapable of work.[50]

It is virtually impossible to open the report at any page without being confronted with details of appalling living conditions, immorality, filthy streets, human neglect and the lack of adequate sanitation and water supplies. Despite his clear view that health was closely linked to living conditions he was devoted to the 'miasmic' theory: that by removing foul smells from the home, the residents' health would be improved.

Even in his final year, 1890, seven years after Robert Koch had identified the cholera bacillus in India, he still held to this view. Just two of the hundreds of examples in the book illustrate some of the above points. In Sleaford, Lincolnshire, he reports on overcrowding and the subsequent intolerable smell, and on the question of the lack of morality in Leeds, as follows:

Eight persons slept in one small ill-ventilated apartment, with scarcely any bed clothing. The vitiated air must have been respired over and over again, by eight individuals. It is not surprising that this family should have been affected by fever.[51]

In the houses of the working classes, brothers and sisters, and lodgers of both sexes, are found occupying the same sleeping room with the parents, and consequences occur which humanity shudders to contemplate.[52]

The housing type and quality varied from town to town but in most of the rapidly growing towns the cellar dwelling and the appalling in-fill that took place in yards and folds, with their tunnel entrances, were the areas of major concern. There was usually a lack of paving that was distasteful to passers by, forced to walk in dust or mud according to the season.[53] For those forced to live in such an area there was also no drainage for rainwater, and street sweeping, often where domestic rubbish accumulated, was virtually impossible. The lack of basic amenities was outlined by Robert Baker in his initial Leeds report of 1839 when he wrote:

It seems to your committee that some of the property where the working classes reside has been laid out without any reference to the erecting of out offices. Thus, for instance, for three streets at the Bank, containing one hundred dwellings and a population of 452 persons, there are but two small offices, neither of which is fit for use, one street being wholly destitute of this provision.[54]

There appeared to be little control over the development of the industrial city and in his book *Housing Problem in England* E. R. Dewsnap cites twenty-eight Public Housing and Public Health Acts between 1851 and 1903 and notes that the recommendations were mainly of a permissive nature. The Nuisances Act of 1855 in recognising overcrowding and its dire consequences on health, had provisions that are dismissed by him as 'nugatory'.[55]

The new developments that were built in towns away from the immediate centres were often of poor quality. One example of the housing being built is the often-maligned back-to-back property. Although no street of back-to-back houses was built in Leeds before 1787, there had been a number of properties built without a back door prior to that time. This style of building was, indicates Beresford, inevitable once cottages began to be built 'backsides' in folds and yards. The length of the yard tempted the insertion, he suggests, of cottage after cottage, as in the notorious Boot and Shoe Yard, replacing such outbuildings as hayloft that lined the walls. The yard had, in fact, two lines of 'blind back' properties, a single room deep.[56]

The back-to-back house was different from much of the housing, such as that in yards, tenements, cellar dwellings and lodging houses, that grew out of the industrial development of towns, in that it was designed for use by a single working-class family. It was essentially, suggests Burnett, the speculative builder's answer to the mass demand for urban working class housing that was economical, easy to build and yet would provide a 'clearly identifiable house' with water and a shared privy. Although condemned almost totally by sanitary reformers, it was still being built in Leeds in 1937.[57]

The outstanding disadvantage of the back-to-back house lay, indicates Burnett, in its lack of amenities. However, by 1886 Leeds had forty-nine thousand such properties constituting 71 per cent of its housing provision, and there were vast numbers in many other northern towns. Following a survey of 3,706 houses in

Halifax by the MOH, for his 1876 report, it was noted that of these 1,997 only had one bedroom, 290 only had one room (in some cases a cellar) for living and sleeping and only ninety had a back and a front or through ventilation. Additionally, 668 had defective privy accommodation.[58] Ranger had already referred to a want of privy accommodation some twenty-years earlier.[59] Eventually 'the preoccupation with privies' led to the development of the through terrace house with light and access at both front and back. The grid-iron system that remains in most towns, with its back alley layout, gave easy access to night soil men.[60] Between 1886 and 1904 two-thirds of all new houses built in Leeds were back-to-back, although a by-law of 1886 had decreed that space should be left every four pairs, in which privies could be erected, or access gained to them.[61]

It is difficult to identify which of the three causes of premature death - inadequate sanitation, overcrowding or poverty - was the most prevalent. Dr. George Gregory, whose lecture was reported in the *Lancet* in April 1843, believed that the greatest foe to health and long life was poverty. Disease did usually find a home in undernourished souls and he believed that 'all descriptions of disease find in them [the undernourished] their chief victims'.[62]

The Diseases

What then were the diseases that the conditions outlined above had a profound effect upon? What were the endemic and epidemic diseases that found a home in the epidemic streets with their many health hazards? The list is, in a sense, endless. In addition to those that provide us with the chapters of this volume - measles, cholera, smallpox, diphtheria, typhoid, typhus, scarlet fever and influenza there was whooping cough, tuberculosis and, closely linked to influenza, pneumonia. When considering deaths of mothers and children infantile diarrhoea and childbed fever should be added to this list. As the table below shows, by the end of the nineteenth century there had been a considerable reduction in deaths from a number of these infectious diseases, especially smallpox, scarlet fever, typhus and typhoid.

Table 1:3   Prevalent disease deaths 1840-1910 from annual reports of the Registrar General [63]

	1840	1850	1860	1870	1880	1890	1900	1910
Smallpox	10,876	4,753	2,882	2,857	651	16	85	19
Typhus*				3,520	611	151	29	5
Typhoid	19,040	15,435	14,084	9,185	7,160	5,148	5,591	1,889
Scarlet Fever	21,377	14,756	10,578	34,628	18,703	6,974	3,844	2,370
Whooping cough	6,352	8,285	8,956	12,528	14,103	13,756	11,467	8,797
Measles	9,566	7,332	9,805	7,986	13,690	12,614	12,710	8,302
Pneumonia	19,083	21,138	26,586	25,147	27,099	40,373	44,300	39,760
Tuberculosis	63,870	50,202	55,345	57,973	51,711	48,366	42,987	36,334

*Typhus and typhoid were not distinguished from each other until 1869

Many of these conditions found a ready home in the filthy streets and insanitary conditions that prevailed. Many were endemic and the population may well have been resigned to these. Many diseases, although appearing in epidemic form locally, never disappeared from annual medical returns. Measles and scarlet fever both fall into this category. The diseases can also be loosely divided into infections that attacked mainly those amongst the poorer classes and those that found a home amongst all classes; typhus and typhoid being good examples of the difference. The former, a louse borne infection, was mainly associated with dirt, poverty and overcrowding, whereas typhoid found its victims in a wide range of homes – even, as we shall hear, in Buckingham Palace. The infections can also be divided even further into those mainly of childhood, such as diphtheria, measles and scarlet fever and those that attacked all ages.

One endemic condition not considered in this book, that Hardy indicates was 'widely felt and widely feared' by all levels of society, was tuberculosis.[64] Although it is a chronic infectious disease, spread by droplets of infected sputum, that rose to prominence as towns expanded, it was not accepted as such until the end of the nineteenth century. In fact it did not attain infectious disease status until 1912. Like typhus, it was associated chiefly with domestic habit, and poorly ventilated, crowded and unhygienic surroundings where the microbe spreads best. It did, though, affect the poorer classes proportionately more than the rich. This was, clearly, not always the case, and in 1875 J.F. Churchill pronounced that 'not only the poor but the rich, the powerful and the promising will be allowed to sink prematurely into the grave'. He indicated that of the hundred thousand suffering from consumption and allied diseases of the tubercular type at that time, sixty thousand would be dead within a year – their places to be filled with an equal number of victims.[65] It was a disease that was also often associated, in a strangely romantic way, with artists and poets. This was, perhaps, simply because the early or relatively early deaths of, for example, John Keats in 1821; Emily Bronte in 1848; Elizabeth Barrett Browning in 1861 and Robert Louis Stevenson in 1894 caught the public's eye. However, as Crawford points out, in reality the disease is far from romantic.[66]

The infection shows itself in different forms and two of these cause disease in man. The human form was responsible for virtually all respiratory (pulmonary) tuberculosis, also referred to as phthisis or consumption, and for 70 per cent of non-pulmonary cases. Bovine tuberculosis, generally transmitted through infected milk, is responsible for the rest of the cases. This was usually associated with the disease in infants and children. At the end of the nineteenth century the disease in all its forms was still responsible for 2,010 deaths per million living. Despite Robert Koch's discovery of the tubercle bacillus in 1882 no treatment for the condition was developed until 1943 when Streptomycin became available.[67]

We will now consider, in chronological order, how these often lethal infectious diseases, in epidemic form, had a profound effect on the lives of nineteenth-century and, in two cases, twentieth-century West Yorkshire. We begin in Leeds in 1809 where the population, although growing, was still around fifty thousand.

Chapter Two

The Fatal Effects of a Malady

Measles in Leeds during 1809 and 1891

Measles is a highly contagious disease that is conveyed by droplets of saliva or by touch. As with other diseases, the risk of infection was increased in the nineteenth century by the prevalence, especially in the rapidly-growing industrial areas, of one-roomed living and by both the healthy and the sick often sharing the same bed.[1] Leeds, like many other industrial towns and indeed smaller communities, experienced a number of measles epidemics. The two that are of interest here occurred some eighty years apart, in 1809 and in 1891. The first epidemic is of particular interest owing to its severity during the summer months; the second one was rather more subtle, and resulted in an enquiry by the Local Government Board.[2] Others of considerable severity were recorded in 1893-4 and 1917-18.

Measles was a major killer in the nineteenth century and by 1807-08 had, in London, overtaken smallpox in the list of bills of mortality. Even today the virus kills around 350,000 children worldwide amongst unvaccinated people.[3] In the United Kingdom there were, for example, only fifty-six confirmed cases in 1998. However, by 2003 that number had increased to 438 and further increases resulted in a total of 739 in 2006. Following an outbreak in Lille and Bordeaux in 2010 parents were urged by the Foreign Secretary, William Hague, to ensure that their children were vaccinated prior to travelling to France. This message was repeated at Easter, 2011.[4] It is generally agreed that the increase is due almost entirely to the scare over the safety of triple vaccines.

Measles was, and indeed still is, extremely virulent when linked to malnutrition. When endemic in Britain it appeared throughout the year but the peak incidence was often during the summer months. There was also a high case-to-mortality rate in the winter, when it was linked to coughs and influenza.[5] The disease was also closely associated with whooping cough with which it often operated in tandem. Whooping cough was the 'poor relation'[6] of childhood disease and although history often links it with measles, it that was a killer in its own right.[7] Creighton believed that whooping cough outbreaks often followed measles but most commentators appear to be less sure about this sequence.[8] A trawl through any school log book often produces evidence of measles outbreaks, and the resultant closures, and in many cases makes clear the link between outbreaks of both measles and whooping cough. The following are from Lightcliffe, near Halifax, but could have been from virtually any school in the nineteenth and early twentieth centuries.

16 November 1894: *Epidemic of measles has broken out in the district. A great number of children are away. The infants' school at Hipperholme is closed for the above reason*

21 November 1894: *Closed the school today owing to the epidemic spreading.*

11 July 1902: *The attendance in the infant school has suffered terribly in the last four weeks from an epidemic of whooping cough and measles.*[9]

It is thought that the disease has been around for approximately 5,000 years in the old world. Measles has, indicates Crawford, 'many relatives' but is most closely linked to the rinderpest virus of cattle.[10] Once cities began to grow, measles took a foothold and in many cases became endemic. In more rural communities it erupted from time to time in epidemic waves. It is a classic 'crowd disease' and in addition to industrial development, the growing development of elementary education in the nineteenth century provided additional reservoirs of infection.[11]

Measles is characterized by a fever with a cough, a runny nose and red eyes before the typical red rash appears over the body. It is a viral infection and remains infectious until the rash begins to fade. It could have been rendered less dangerous in the past by a system of early notification and isolation but this was clearly not the case in many nineteenth-century households. Poor parents tended to be stoical about the disease and appear not to have even sought free medical advice from, for example, a dispensary.[12] Mortality rates varied in relation to the severity of the disease and the general health of the victim. Those, as indicated, who lived in crowded conditions, were undernourished, and were not given access to even basic medical care were at the greatest risk. The proportion of deaths to attacks was far lower amongst those who were better off.[13] The chance of a child, for it was children who accounted for virtually all measles' deaths, dying from diarrhoea associated with the disease was particularly high. Complications associated with the disease, in addition to diarrhoea, include pneumonia, damage to the nervous system, encephalitis and occasionally blindness. The hunt for a successful vaccine had begun in the mid eighteenth century but, unlike Edward Jenner's smallpox vaccine, Scottish physician Francis Home's procedure did not 'catch on'. It was not, in fact, until 1963 that the first live-attenuated measles vaccine was licensed.[14] As was the case with many of the diseases we shall discuss there was, unsurprisingly, a wide range of quack remedies and palliative treatment on offer across the centuries, including the inevitable enemas. I would, therefore, have been disappointed if I had not come across the following advice, in relation to measles, in the first addition of Pears' Cyclopaedia:[15]

The principal points to attend to in the treatment of the disease are to see that the bowels are evacuated everyday.

There was, co-incidentally, similar advice offered in relation to those suffering from scarlet fever when it was considered necessary to 'keep the bowels freely moved every day'.[16]

It appears to be clear, however, that none of the preventative measures aimed at measles, and indeed the other infectious diseases of childhood, were in any way successful in changing their behaviour during the nineteenth and early twentieth centuries.[17] This view was supported by Dr. B.A. Whitelegge, the County Medical Officer for the West Riding of Yorkshire on 21 December 1892, when speaking to the London Epidemiological Society. Although advancing knowledge had provided better means of health protection, 'measles and whooping cough have, as yet, shown little tendency to diminish their ravages'.[18]

Finally, and by way of further introduction to the Leeds epidemics, it may be interesting to look at the national picture in relation to mortality rates during the nineteenth century. Registration of deaths began, as we have seen, during the second half of 1837 and William Farr, to all intents and purposes the first Registrar-General for England and Wales, presented his first report in 1839. He claimed that this provided 98 per cent coverage but Smith believes that this was an over ambitious figure and indicates that, for example, initially many illegitimate live births, and deaths of premature babies went unrecorded.[19] Even if the figures produced are somewhat underestimated, they still provide an excellent guide to Victorian measles mortality rates. From the first full year of available statistics for the disease in 1838 until the end of the century the annual number of recorded deaths from measles in England and Wales only once fell below the 5,000 mark (in 1853) and in the other years passed 10,000 twenty-two times. In 1887 the figure was 16,765. The annual figure was still over 9,000 at the outbreak of the First World War in 1914.[20]

The 1809 Epidemic

This outbreak was so severe that the *Leeds Mercury* announced on 17 June 1809 that:

We have cautiously abstained from mentioning the mortality produced by the measles in this town, within the last three months, from a fear of augmenting the alarm so naturally created by the fatal effects of that malady.[21]

The following chart (see table 2:1) was, however, published in the paper on 17 June 1809, giving the weekly numbers of interments at the Parish Church. Between 1 March and 31 May of that year there had been 491 funerals at the Parish Church and 230 of these were related to the burial of measles' victims. April and May were the months that saw the epidemic at its most aggressive, with 233 deaths. The reminder of the deaths were from what the paper described as 'the great variety of miscellaneous complaints incident on mankind'.

The end of May did not though, by any means, herald the end of the epidemic and it was not until 15 October that the last victims of this fearsome outbreak, Henry Parker aged fifteen months, of Kendall Row, and George Knowling aged fourteen months, of Hunslet Lane, were buried. The strength of the epidemic had subsided somewhat by the end of August but deaths linked, I suggest, to the same outbreak, continued to occur at regular intervals. The winter saw no burials of measles' victims and the first death attributed to the disease in 1810 was that of twenty-two months old Nathaniel Ramsden, of Marsh Lane on 6 May.

Table 2:1 Weekly list of funerals at the Leeds Parish Church in Leeds March-May 1809

		Measles	Other			Measles	Other
March	1-8	2	15	April	18-26	23	22
March	8-15	5	18	April/May	26-3	35	11
March	15-22	4	19	May	3-10	31	25
March	22-29	9	13	May	10-17	35	22
March/April	29-5	19	14	May	17-24	22	28
April	5-11	24	12	May	24-31	18	11
April	11-18	29	22	Totals		261	230

Unlike, say, the Denby Dale outbreak of typhoid (chapter nine), there is no clear starting point to an epidemic such as this. However, it is possible from burial records to see a pattern developing and to identify the early victims. The first victims of the epidemic, that began slowly, were William the son of James Ogden of Kirkgate, and William the son of Achsah Day, of Off Street that was situated to the south of York Street and adjacent to Duke Street. They were buried on 28 February 1809, aged fifteen months and ten months respectively.

The number of deaths increased to thirty-one during March with homes in York Street, Duke Street, Quarry Hill and Marsh Lane being affected during the first two weeks.[22] Clearly at this stage the infection was confined to an area to the east of the town and a look at a contemporary map (see figure 2:1) will indicate how these streets were the main arteries running through, or embracing, this part of Leeds. This was an area with poor housing, confined yards and limited fresh air and sanitation. Many of these appalling yards were named after their owners and were only accessible via narrow and dingy tunnels. The Bank, an area situated to the east of Marsh Lane and the south of York Road, was a particularly crowded district of mean houses. Even before the population explosion of the 1840s, when suddenly there were eleven thousand people living there in just eleven acres, manufacturers had been attracted to the area by the local coal deposits, water from the river and cheap land.[23]

Although the epidemic did eventually spread beyond this confined area, as we shall see, when the final figures are considered it will be noted that many of the addresses that show the highest mortality rates are those where the measles first found a home. The first sign that the disease was spreading beyond the original confined area was recorded on 19 April with the death of Richard Micklethwaite of Bridge (Leeds Bridge). The virus was about to cross the river and it arrived in Hunslet Lane about a week later. Burials of those living in that lane followed and by early May it was in Meadow Lane. Before the end of the month addresses on Water Lane and in Holbeck had been struck.

Although deaths occurred throughout the epidemic in these areas, the disease never really established a foothold and no more than twenty deaths were recorded

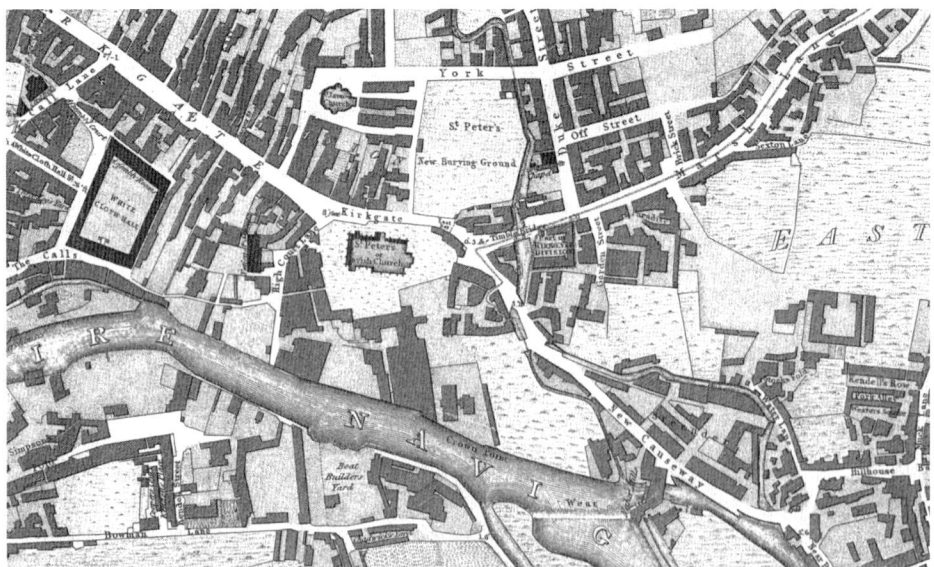

Figure 2:1 The area where the first outbreaks occurred in February 1809
From *A Plan of the Town of Leeds and its Environs 1815*. Netlam and Frances Giles
(The Thoresby Society)

in homes south of the River Aire. The disease also established itself in Briggate to the west but again surprisingly, considering the number of confined areas there, was not especially lethal; and briefly to Mabgate in the north east, where nine died, in late July. The greatest number of measles deaths, seventy-four, was recorded as being in Bank; Kirkgate saw thirty-three; Quarry Hill, twenty-three; Ebenezer Street, twenty-two and Marsh Lane, twenty. The workhouse recorded fifteen deaths.

The epidemic began to gather pace during April when 115 died of measles. On 23 April eleven victims of the epidemic were buried. One of the victims was four years old, one three years and the rest two or younger. On the same day five others were buried. One of these, a child of two, was a victim of smallpox, the others were adults aged seventy-two, thirty-eight, twenty-four and twenty-three. The cause of death is given as 'decline' for the three youngest adults. No cause is given for the death of Mary Dixon, the eldest. In May the total number of measles victims rose again, to 117, after which there was a marked fall to thirty-nine in June and nineteen in July. The final two victims of the outbreak were, as we have heard, buried on 15 October.

Inevitably, it is possible to see from the registers that some families suffered greatly during the epidemic with more than one death occurring in a short space of time. In May, William Gardner and his wife buried three of their children within a period of four days. William aged three years and Mary Ann, one, on 7 May and Jane aged five three days later. An identical situation arose in the household of Thomas Brooks, a soldier in the forty-fourth foot regiment billeted in Leeds. On 14 April he buried John, aged three years, and Thomas aged nine months; and three days later, James his four year-old son. There are many examples of two children from the same family being interred at the same time. One of the more unusual examples

The Fatal Effects of a Malady

concerned the Cooper family when two sons, Matthew and John, were buried on 20 April. John was almost seven years older than his brother and at eight years one of the oldest children on the register.

Table 2:2 The ages of 312 measles victims recorded in St Peter's Church burial register: February-July 1809. It will be noted that an overwhelming number of victims were under the age of two.

Age	Number	Percentage	Age	Number	Percentage
Under one	49	15.7	Seven	1	0.3
One	93	29.8	Eight	5	1.5
Two	81	25.9	Eleven	2	0.6
Three	42	13.4	Thirteen	1	0.3
Four	16	5.1	Sixteen	1	0.3
Five	18	5.7	Twenty-three	1	0.3
Six	10	3.2	Seventy-nine*	1	0.3

* This was William Dinsley of Long Balk Lane who was buried 16 May.

It may now be interesting to consider some of the other deaths recorded in the burial register. As we have seen, of the 491 funerals at the Parish Church during

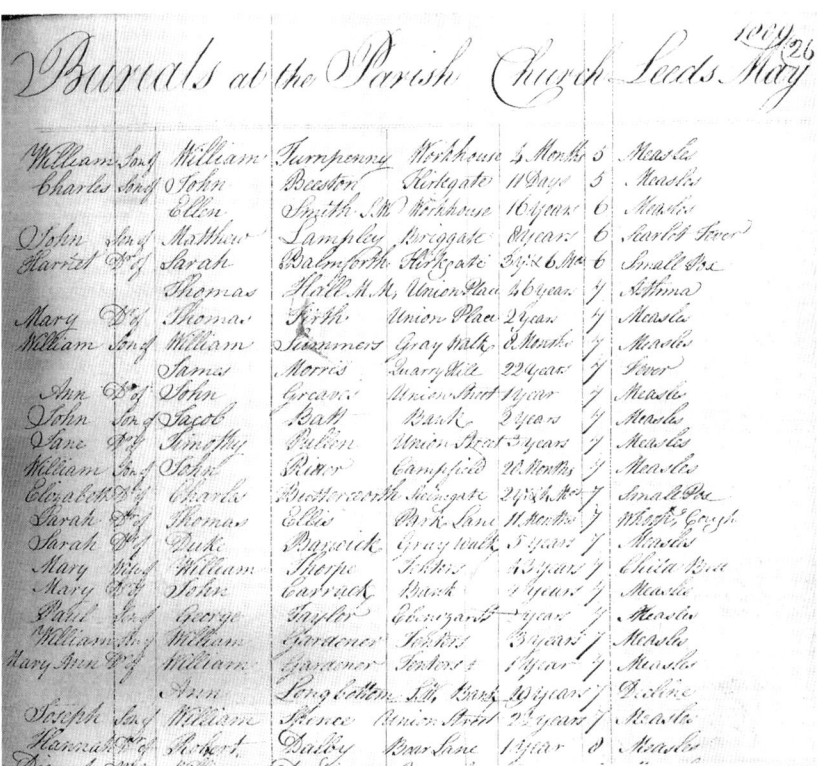

Figure 2:2 St. Peter's Church burial register, May 1809
(West Yorkshire Archives, Leeds. Ref: RDP68/2/88)

17

these months, 261 (53 per cent) were 'occasioned by measles alone' and the rest were from the great variety of miscellaneous complaints. What were these complaints? Many and varied is the easy answer, with a marked inclination towards 'decline'. In fact, fifty-nine of the 230 other deaths were the result of this condition. Other 'popular' causes of death during March, April and May were whooping cough (16) fits (21) and, although it never approached epidemic form, smallpox (30). A random sampling of the registers for other causes produces, for example, inflammation of the bowels, worms, inflammation of the lungs, teeth, bleeding cansey, ague, water in the brain, mortification, and old age. The youngest person to fall into the latter category was sixty-nine years old; the eldest (by far) was Ann Shann, a widow of Meadow Lane, who died at the remarkable age of ninety-five.

The 1809 measles epidemic had a devastating effect on a small section of the Leeds community. Little could be done to quell its deadly journey from house to house through the yards in Kirkgate, Quarry Hill and Bank area. Measles, as we have seen, continued to break out in homes across the British Isles for more than a century after this epidemic. What became clear over the years was that, as B. A. Whitelegge said in 1892, 'each recurring outbreak finds the same sort of population as the last'.[24] This becomes increasingly clear as we go forward seventy-two years, almost three generations, to 1891 and consider the measles epidemic that caused many fatalities in a short period of time and baffled the authorities.

The 1891 Outbreak

Outbreaks in Leeds were common. However, in 1891 an outbreak in two of the Leeds districts resulted in 'exceptional mortality', and a published report at the request of the Local Government Board. The report was written by the Medical Officer of Health, Dr. J. Spottiswoode Cameron.[25] There had been a similar request following a severe outbreak in 1886 when there had been 193 deaths. During the following three years the deaths amounted to 206, 197 and 339 respectively. These figures, when set against the population, were said by the MOH in 1890 to indicate that 'in this respect we resemble most large towns'. What appeared to be of particular interest now was the fact that the 1891 outbreak was particularly severe during the first quarter of the year in just two of the Borough's registration sub-districts : North Leeds and South-East Leeds , where there had been a total of 123 deaths. The ninety in North Leeds corresponded to a mortality rate of 5.95 (per 1000 per annum) and the thirty-three in South-East Leeds to a rate of 3.96. The measles death rate for that year in the whole borough was 1.87.

Why was it then that only two districts, those immediately to the north and south of York Road, were attacked so severely? This was the question that the MOH had to address to satisfy his masters in London. To begin with he simply recorded the the ages of the victims and the type of housing where the deaths occurred. (see table 2:3)

He then decided to approach his report by dividing the houses where measles struck - mildly or fatally into two categories: 'death houses' and 'recovery houses'. No deaths occurred in properties classified as 'recovery houses' but some patients did recover in 'death houses'. These houses were then divided into two groups: back to back or 'salt-pie' (blind back) houses formed one group, through houses the other. (See table 2:4)

Table 2:3 Fatality figures for the north and south-east of the Borough during January-March 1891.

Ages:	0-1	1-5	15-25	Housing: Back-to-back	Through
North	18	64	8	77	13
South-East	4	25	4	29	4

In the death houses 84.9 per cent had no through ventilation, whereas in the recovery houses the percentage of houses without a through draft was 76 per cent. The death houses also had marginally more occupants per room. (1.88 to 1.72) but this difference was barely significant. The table below also shows the sanitary condition in the two categories of houses. The final category, covering such matters as general cleanliness, did not include 'closet arrangement' as this was considered separately. A long and complicated section was devoted to trough closets, privy middens and water closets and my conclusion is that some of the evidence here was both contradictory and inconclusive.

Table 2:4 The sanitary arrangements in Measles 'death-houses and 'recovery-houses' for the thirteen weeks ended 4 April 1891.

	Back to back or 'salt-pie'	Through	Persons per room	Drainage and cleanliness. Good	Bad
Death-houses	84.9%	15.1%	1.88	12.8%	87.2%
Recovery-houses	76.0%	24.0%	1.72	16.0%	84.0%

It is difficult to know just what the Local Government Board, or the reader, would have gleaned from Dr. Cameron's report. His final paragraphs draw much of the information together and it is clear that such factors as isolation could have had some effect on the spread of the disease. It was, however, in his view a moot point whether closing schools, so popular at the time, had as much effect as was thought. He indicates that 'the children instead of being at school, are in the streets, and are mixing freely with members of the infected families'. Dr. Cameron was also firmly convinced that, until he and others could educate the public that measles was an 'unnecessary disease', and that 'if mothers could postpone the attack in their children until they are older and therefore have greater chances of recovery', any measures would have little chance of succeeding. This view is supported by the figures from the 172 fatal cases across Leeds where 92 per cent of the deaths had occurred in children five years old or younger. Only four per cent of children under the age of one year had recovered compared with 61 per cent of those attacked between the ages of one and five.[26]

What then are our conclusions and why were only the two areas badly affected?

From a distance of over 100 years it does seem to be reasonably clear that living conditions, which are also often linked to levels of poverty, over-crowding and malnutrition, are again factors closely related to the mortality rates. An example of some of the conditions favouring illness can be found in the 1893 Leeds MOH report that analyses the deaths of 153 children under the age of one, many often within a few weeks of birth, during a six-week period in the autumn. The following information, taken from that report, makes harrowing reading:

Mother diarrhoea. Artificially fed. (Died aged sixteen days)
Artificially fed. Bottle not scalded. House crowded. (One month)
Dirty WC. Pool in yard from neighbours' closet. (Two months)
Fed artificially Swiss milk and sugar. Bottle not sterilized. (Three months)
Wasting and diarrhoea from birth. Mother had p.[peurperal] fever. (Four months)
Wasting from birth. Mother consumptive. (Five months)
Fed milk (unboiled) and 'ordinary food'. (Eight months)

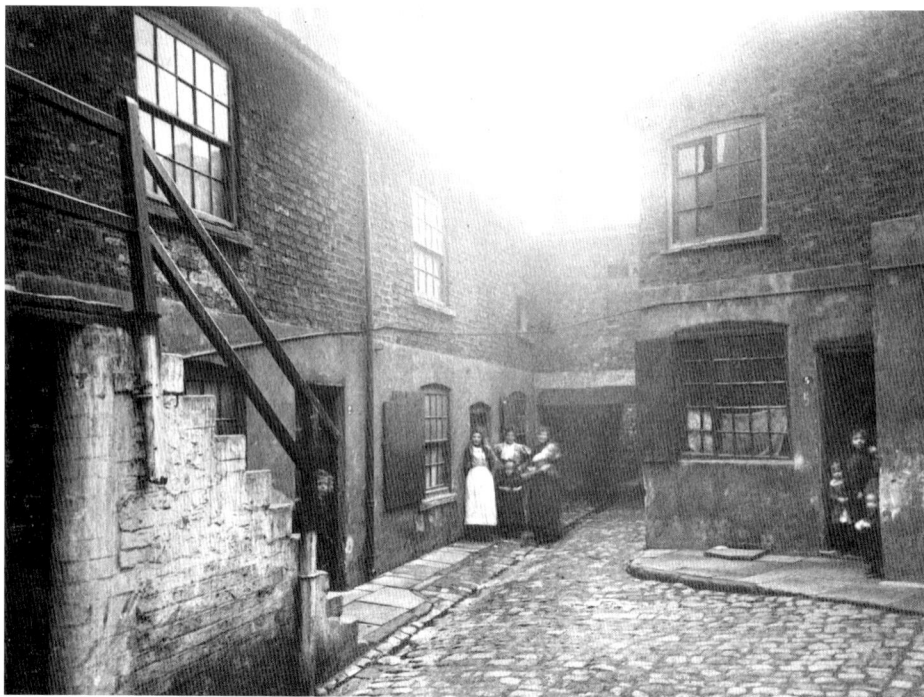

Figure 2:3 Marsh Lane Court off Marsh Lane, 1901. Many of the victims lived in cramped and unhealthy yards such as this. (See also figure 2.4)
(Leeds Library and Information Services. www.leodis.net)

The two areas of Leeds badly affected in 1891 were the ones with the highest population density and some of the poorest housing conditions. The medical profession had already, as indicated, accepted that the proportion of deaths to attacks was far lower amongst the wealthy classes than amongst the poorer, or even artisan classes. [27] 1891 was not by any means the end of measles outbreaks of considerable severity in the city. In 1893-4, 630 people fell victim to the diseases prey and in 1917-18, 694. [28] In his report of 1918, when influenza was killing so many people in the city (256 alone in one week ending 9 November), the MOH still reminded his readers that:

Measles as a killing disease is of vastly greater importance to the community than scarlet fever, diphtheria, enteric fever either singly or taken together. During an epidemic it attacks practically all the susceptibles.[29]

However, the final word perhaps should rest with B.A. Whitelegge who finished the address to which we have already referred with the following salutary remark:

I have no explanation to offer as to the causes which bring about these major epidemics[30]

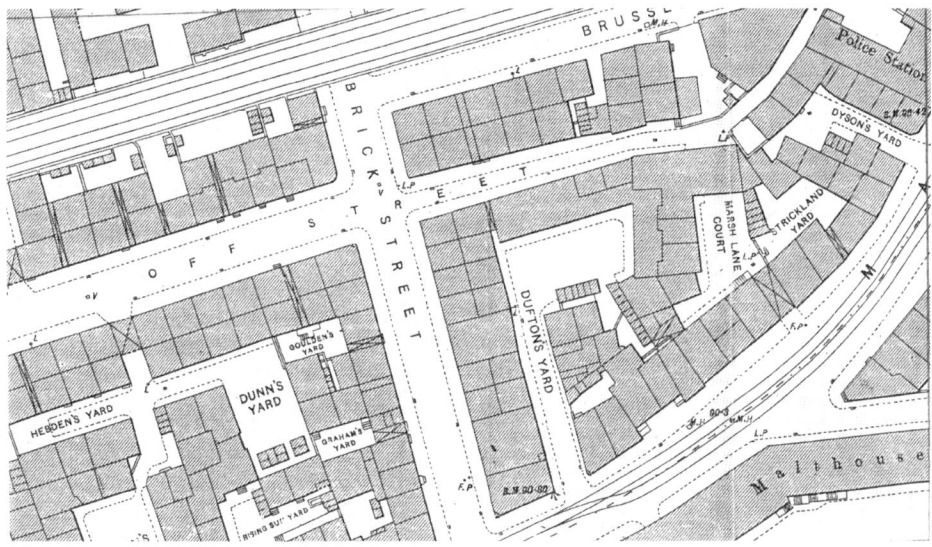

Figure 2:4 Marsh Lane Court
(Ordnance Survey, 1891. Sheet CCXVIII. Original scale 1:500.)

The location of Marsh Lane Court, one of many such yards off Marsh Lane. Also seen here are Dufton's Yard (front cover) and Goulden's Yard (Chapter four)

Chapter Three

A Tidal Wave of Disease

The 1832 Leeds Cholera Epidemic

The Pestilence Extends to Leeds

On Thursday 5 April 1832 a small but chilling news item appeared in the *Leeds Intelligencer*. It informed the 76,000 people of Leeds that cholera had broken out in Goole and that several deaths had occurred. It was now clear, the paper indicated, that 'the pestilence has gained a footing in Yorkshire'.[1] This news was to provide a direct link with the Leeds cholera epidemic that was to claim 702 lives, lead to accusations of medical malpractice and provoke local disturbances.

The port of Goole is situated some forty miles to the east of Leeds and although the railway link between the two towns did not open until 1848 (it had reached Selby, a half way mark, in 1834)[2] there was a strong commercial link via the waterways. In April the cholera had begun to spread inland from Hull, where the epidemic was causing particular concern as fifteen people had died from the disease, following the Humber estuary and the river Ouse[3] to Goole, Selby and Market Weighton. It then spread along the Aire and Calder navigation to Leeds. Wandering tribes that fulfilled the needs of the British economy for manual labour in the countryside and the towns also acted as major transmitters of cholera. An additional, but unwelcome, guest on their travels was, suggests Durey, *vibrio cholerae*.[4] Vagrants, like the wandering tribes, were also 'on tramp' via the footpaths linking Goole with the West.[5]

On 14 April it was reported that, 'no vessel was to leave Goole for the West without a clean bill of health'.[6] However, there were still overland coach links from Goole to Liverpool, London, York and Hull.

Leeds had, initially, received notice of the cholera threat in October 1831 when news arrived from Sunderland that on 27 October Dr. James Butler Kell had had the 'melancholy task' of reporting the death from cholera of William Sproat an inhabitant of the town.[7] It was on the 23 of October that Sproat, a keelman, had begun his 'short but disastrous contribution to British medical history'. On that day he became ill with violent vomiting and purging, cramps of the stomach and other associated symptoms, and three days later he was dead. Sproat was the first confirmed victim of Asiatic cholera in the British Isles.[8] The North Sea had clearly not prevented the disease that had been raging in Europe, and was identified in

Hamburg on 12 October, from arriving in the North East of England. It was then that the Mayor of Leeds, William Hey, resolved to form the Leeds Board of Health to deal with any subsequent outbreak. The board was to consist of town magistrates, the vicar of Leeds, physicians and surgeons of the infirmary, the dispensary and the house of recovery plus some of the town's principal inhabitants. Thirteen separate districts or divisions were to facilitate the board's work,[9] with a medical man in charge of each.[10] However, there was little optimism exuding from the board's sub-committee as it was reported in the Intelligencer that:

Should any contagious disorder fix itself amongst this dense population, its spread would defy the utmost exertions of medical staff[11]

Cholera was something of a shock disease and had, according to Wohl, an impact out of all proportion to its statistical importance. Its effect was both quick and lethal and it carried with it a high percentage of fatalities amongst those contracting the disease. The victim could often be dead within hours. The symptoms included violent stomach pains, vomiting, diarrhoea and total prostration during which the body turned cold and blue, the eyes and cheeks sunken and the skin wizened. The 'blue phase' usually indicated that death was imminent. Of all these the major symptom was the explosive diarrhoea that produced what Gill and Holland have termed 'hugely voluminous stools' that have an appearance of yellowish water. They are often referred to as rice water stools as they contain evidence of the lining of the intestines.[12]

The first deaths in Yorkshire had in fact occurred at Doncaster as early as 7 January 1832. Two sailors had arrived in the town the previous evening of 6 January after visiting Hull, Leeds and Wakefield. One of them died the following morning from symptoms 'very suspicious' of Asiatic cholera. Outbreaks in Hull had followed but the disease does not appear to have taken on epidemic proportions at that time.[13] When the *Leeds Mercury* reported on 15 May that the disease had reached Selby many began to realise that the great tidal wave of cholera was now almost upon

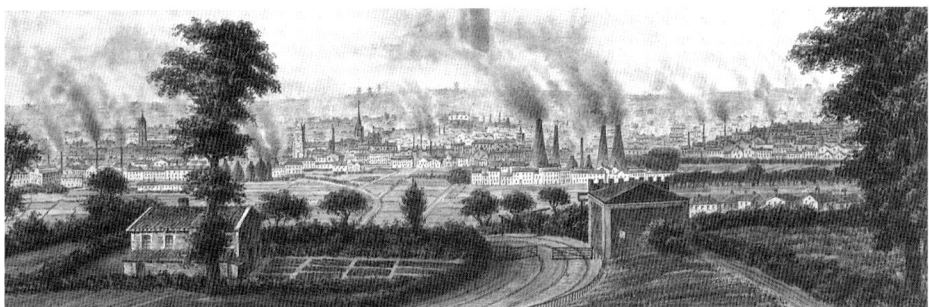

Figure 3:1 Leeds from Rope-Hill, South Leeds c 1840.
(Thoresby Society MS 39B32)

Drawn by Alphonse Douseau from 'a hill called Rope-Hill', Middleton. Leeds Pottery is to the left below Trinity Church. To the centre right the conical chimneys of Hunslet glass works can be seen and on the far right the mills of the Bank. Plumes of smoke 'rise like fumaroles over some volcanic plane'.[14]

them.[15] It had travelled to Selby via a boatman, Thomas Hughes aged twenty-one, who from 28 April had spent several days ferrying vagrants across the Ouse for York races.[16] His case, suggests Underwood, presents an interesting exercise in epidemiological speculation. On 2 May Hughes was stricken with cholera but recovered. However, within eleven days his brother, father, uncle John Kendle (whom he visited the day that he was first taken ill), and his cousin were attacked. A resident, John Graves, of the same court as Hughes, was also attacked, as was Graves's wife a week later. As Graves and his wife used the same privy 'into which the evacuations of the Hughes family were cast', Underwood believed that it was difficult to see how some common factor could be avoided.[17]

Around two weeks later, on 28 May, cholera had reached Leeds. The first victim was the two year old son of an Irish woollen weaver. The family lived in a small cottage with a single upper room in Blue Bell Fold, a 'small and dirty cul-de-sac' housing twenty poor families, in an area known as Bank.[18] It had long since, notes Beresford, ceased to be a farmyard for folding animals.[19] The fold was situated on the north side of the river Aire in an angle between it and an 'offensive beck or streamlet'[20] and access was gained to by a small alley.[21] The disease spread quickly. Shortly afterwards the boy's young friend died, and several others around the fold fell victim to it.[22]

The disease soon began to radiate outwards. By 7 June it was in Kirkgate and the following day in Quarry Hill. It travelled along York Street to the village of Knostrop and it was in Hunslet and Holbeck by the middle of the month.[23] On 6 June the Board of Health had had no alternative but to declare publicly that cholera was indeed in the town. Their message published on 14 June was clear and, no doubt, confirmed what many already knew:

It is our painful duty to express our decided opinion that the disease called spasmodic cholera has extended to this town. [24]

By the end of July there had been 427 cases and 187 proved to be fatal. This number was to increase considerably during the following months. Not all the cases were reported in the papers but a few caught the editor's eye and were deemed to be worthy of wider coverage. One desperate case from the Boot and Shoe Yard was reported in considerable detail. On 12 June, John Simmonds, a beggar, was attacked with continual purging and other symptoms of the disease. He had no clothes to cover him, no bed to lie on and nothing whatever to eat or drink. His son, also called John, had died two days earlier and his daughter Eve died two days after her brother on the day their father was attacked. His wife and remaining child were apparently starving to death. The dwelling of another victim in the yard was reported, as indicated in the introductory chapter, to be 'abominably, filthy, stinking and destitute'.[25]

The Boot and Shoe Yard, and the adjacent Royal Oak Yard, with their grim blind back tenements abutting the yard walls, were just two of many such yards, especially off Kirkgate, in the town at that time.[26] Their names were usually linked to the inn, or the name of the proprietor of the property, that fronted the yard.[27]

Many, as indicated, were also referred to as folds, or garths, and although technically there was a difference in their origins, the words were usually interchangeable.[28] Yard and fold developments were clearly popular with landlords as they were economical, with their high densities and the absence of water and sanitation. The proprietors, such as John Dufton, who owned many of the houses in the Boot and Shoe Yard, were not charged with the responsibility for paving and drainage as the houses were sited behind the main thoroughfares.[29]

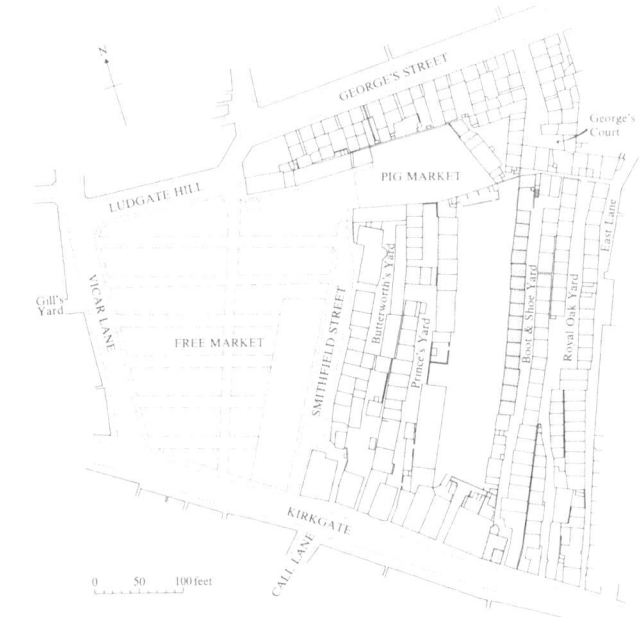

Figure 3:2 The Boot and Shoe Yard in 1843.
(M. Beresford, in D Fraser(Ed), A History of Modern Leeds).

The area surrounding the Boot and Shoe Yard prior to demolition of the properties for the market extension in 1843. The blind back houses that have been crammed into yards and their narrow entrances, often tunnels, can be clearly seen. In this plan the houses of proprietor John Dufton have been shaded.[30]

The towns and cities of Yorkshire had, as we have seen, following the industrial revolution, grown rapidly. Leeds's population had increased by 47.2% during the decade from 1821.[31] Many of these places were amongst the most unsanitary in the country. Pride of place was, however, awarded to Leeds![32] Half the population lived in streets where there was neither sewerage nor cleansing. The Boot and Shoe Yard was but one example, but what an example it was. Few places in the town were so likely to generate disease as this receptacle of poverty, misery and uncleanness, said the *Leeds Mercury*.[33] Here was to be found some of the worst housing in Leeds. The houses here were not only small, some five yards by five yards with one ground floor and one upper floor, but lacked sunlight and ventilation. As the houses had been crowded into the inn yard by lining its inner walls, the front and only door faced inwards to the yard as did any windows. The yard was the home of 340 people who lived approximately ten to a house. There was no water within a quarter of a mile, and only three privies. During the epidemic seventy cart loads of manure that had accumulated over thirty years, were removed from the yard.[34]

Robert Baker's Report

Much of the information relating to the Leeds outbreak is contained in the report of Dr. Robert Baker, dated 3 January 1833. Baker was, at that time, a District Surgeon to the Leeds Board of Health. He was born in York, the second son of John and Hannah on 15 August 1803. He commenced practice in Leeds in 1825, after completing his medical studies at Guy's Hospital, and soon secured a leading position as town surgeon.[35] The following year he was involved in what could have become a minor scandal involving 'resurrection men'. (An incident discussed later in the chapter).[36] In 1833 he took an active part in the Factory Act and was one of the first to realise the need for a system of inspection and supervision in the interests of mill workers. By 1840 the problem of accidents in factories was attracting greater attention and Baker was involved both nationally and locally in the move to reduce the number of accidents in factories. He presented figures from Leeds infirmary in 1840 giving details of accidents happening within Leeds, and the townships of Holbeck and Hunslet. During the year thirty-three patients were admitted and eleven had a limb, foot or digit removed.[37]

He was also compiling a further telling report on the condition of Leeds, around this time. Published in 1842 *On the State and Condition of the Town of Leeds in*

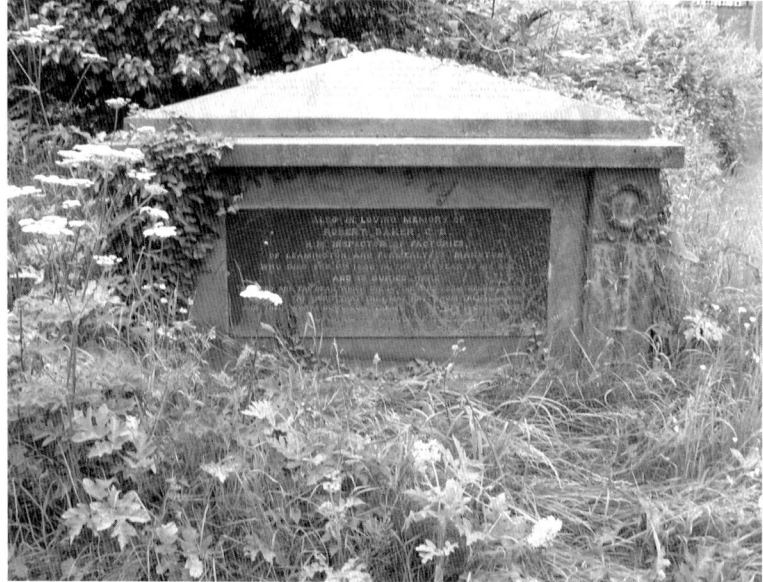

Figure 3:3 Robert Baker's grave in York Cemetery

The epitaph on the family grave notes that Robert Baker C.B, H.M. Inspector of Factories, was a resident of Leamington Spa and formerly of Manston.

the West Riding of the County of York provided not just the Leeds Board with a clear picture of the task before them.[38] It proved, additionally, to be a valuable aid to Edwin Chadwick who indicated that a frightful picture of the condition of the sewerage and drainage in the town was 'afforded to the labouring population.'[39] In 1858 Baker became Inspector of factories for the West of England, Wales and Ireland on behalf of the Home secretary. This area contained 23,346 factories. After retirement, his obituary notes, he enjoyed a 'comparatively short repose from his labours' and died in Leamington Spa on 6 February, 1880, aged seventy-six. Robert Baker is buried in York cemetery.[40]

In his 1833 report to the Board, Baker has much to say about the living conditions and the link between the state of the town and the spread of the disease. The larger part of what is known colloquially as the 'Baker Report' deals with the unpaved streets and yards and the part that they played in the epidemic. In addition to his condemnation of the Boot and Shoe Yard he comments on many other areas. His language is clear and hard hitting as the following examples of filthy streets, taken from the report, make clear:

Bridge Street-In a most filthy state
Baxter's Yard-most dingy, privies open
Cherry Tree Yard-open privies, very bad
Jack Lane-an offensive ditch nearby
Orange Street-most wretchedly bad
Micklethwaite's Yard-stones have to be put down to walk
 Marsh Lane Back-most filthy [41]

He also grades the 586 streets in the town and Underwood has produced figures showing that 247 were classified as 'good', 108 as 'middling', 135 as 'bad' and ninety-six as 'very bad'. The classification 'good' should, indicates Underwood, be taken with reservation as only seventy of those streets belonged to the town.[42]

In a further example he quotes three parallel streets housing 386 persons where there were but two privies. Both were 'totally unusable'. Many of these buildings also contained cellar dwellings 'to boot' and this he suggested was by no means an uncommon occurrence. It was not, though, just the folds and yards that were breeding grounds for the disease. Many victims lived in the back to back housing that lined the grim streets of large sections of the town and there were, for example, eighteen deaths in Quarry Hill, eleven in Richmond Road and eight in York Street.[44] Fleece Lane, where there was a vast mound of night-soil covering an area of some forty square yards, provided a 'striking monument' to civic neglect.[45]

He noted that 755 of the cases during the epidemic occurred in streets that were lacking sewerage and paving. The report, believe Burrell and Gill, provides a fascinating insight into the impact of cholera in Leeds and is, they suggest, 'one of the finest pieces of epidemiology of its time'.[46] Baker carefully mapped the cholera cases, and his work predates that of John Snow who, in 1854, mapped cases in London that he linked to the Broad Street pump.[47] The map, which is attached to the report, shows that the outbreak of the disease was higher in the north and

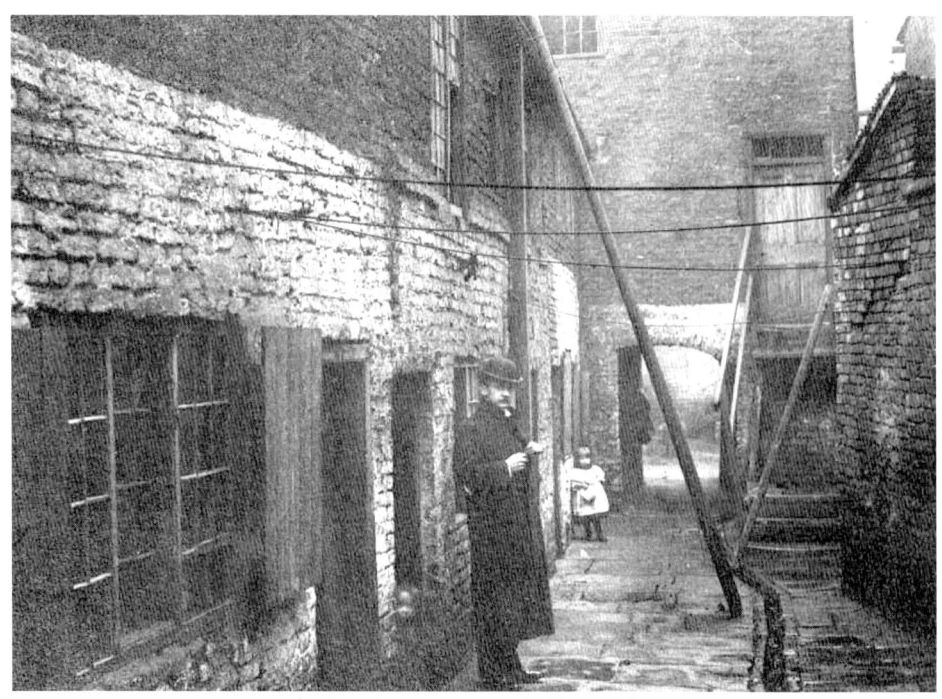

Figure 3:4 The Cherry Tree Yard off 57 Kirkgate, 1901
(Leeds Library and Information Services. www.leodis.net)

Photographed prior to demolition under the Local Government slum clearance programme. The man in the photograph is one of the surveyors who appear on many such photographs of the city's slums. Robert Baker, some seventy years earlier, had identified this partially paved dismal yard, with its narrow entrance and open privies, as one of the many undesirable and 'very bad' yards in the city. Seven of its residents died from cholera during the epidemic. [43]

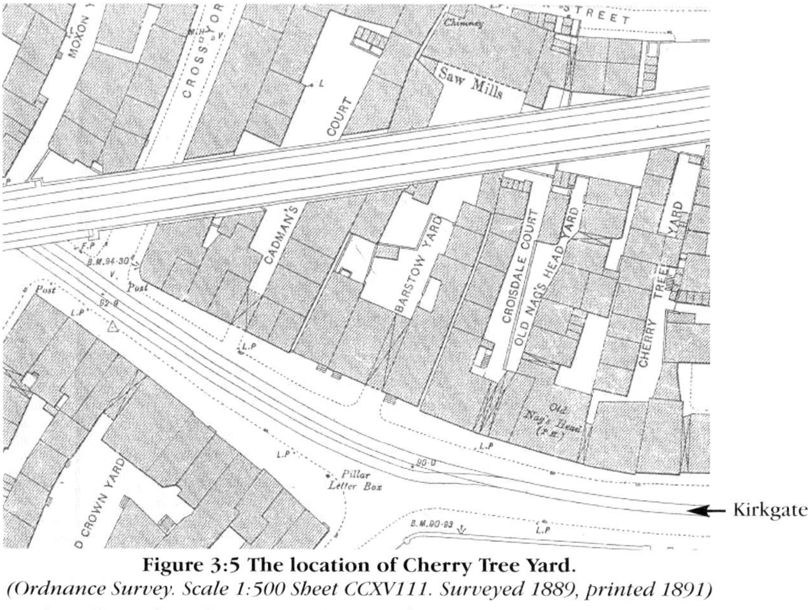

Figure 3:5 The location of Cherry Tree Yard.
(Ordnance Survey. Scale 1:500 Sheet CCXVIII. Surveyed 1889, printed 1891)
The Leeds-Selby railway line opened in 1834 is shown to the north of the yard.

north-east part of the town where the population was denser.[48]

Unlike Snow, however, Baker was never able to identify that the disease was water borne. He did though, Smith suggests, stumble across the relationship between water and cholera, a vibrio-micro organism, without fully understanding its significance.[49] He quotes the example given by Baker when reporting that the disease occurred in the first storey of a building that was occupied by several families he noted that the matter ejected by the victims was thrown down the sink into a sump hole. Here he suggested were two sources of epidemy for those living below, the sump hole and the ejected matter.[50] Underwood argues, however, that Baker had no idea that the poison might be taken into the system through the drinking water and cites the above case as an example.[51] It is also noticeable that the map produced by Baker shows the link between the outbreaks and the many small streams that intersected the infected areas. The streams were for many of the poorer people, their only supply of water for their daily needs. Those living at the higher level took their water from the boreholes, water carriers and local reservoirs. Although the water from the latter would not be acceptable today, as it was pumped from the river, it was considerably cleaner than that from the local becks.[52] Convinced of his miasma theory, perhaps Baker was blinded by his own convictions. Speaking of the direct contact that was proved between the two children who were the first victims, Baker says that:

This would have looked something like contagion, had it not happened that in the course of the week three cases occurred in individuals at a considerable distance from the Blue Bell Fold, where there had been no connection with the former families. [53]

It was not, however, Baker's intention to discuss, he said, the difference of opinion that existed among medical men as to the contagious or epidemic nature of the disease. He was clearly attracted to the miasmic theory and drew the Board's attention to the fact that the disease prevailed in the parts of the town where 'from want of local cleanliness and ventilation, a malignant state of atmosphere was likely to obtain'. Not everybody in properties where the disease was present was a victim and he was keen to stress that those living at a 'higher level' in properties appeared to escape the miasma.[54] He draws also on the experience of the work of Sir John Pringle who produced a treatise on diseases in the army. At a typical camp, the privies and foul straw produced a 'pent and vitiated atmosphere'. In Leeds such a 'condition of the atmosphere' could arise, he believed, in the thousands of stagnant and exhalant surfaces.[55]

We have already seen the condition of the town that is included in the report: The fetid water courses 'corrupted in by both animal and putrefactive matter', the appalling living conditions and the filthy streets. Baker compares Briggate, which was sewered, paved and cleansed, with Kirkgate, although he admits this comparison may not be fair as Kirkgate was in a lower situation and the inhabitants a 'shade lower in condition'[56]

He outlines his findings in relation to the foul air theory and asks why, following his mapping, those 'situated higher' were not affected where the miasma does not exist and proper attention is paid to ventilation and hygiene. He uses many examples from other countries to support his view and could have 'enumerated other corroborative' instances in addition to those he used. He had, though, made out a case that was sufficiently strong to justify the presumption that:

Whether the disease be sporadical, epidemical or endemical-whatever may be the secrete cause there is evidence before this Board of the condition of some parts of the town of Leeds in which it may be latently maintained[57]

Although Baker's miasma theory was 'wildly incorrect' the solution that it offered was to remove the filth from which the smells exuded and did, eventually, reduce the risk of infection, at least in the short term, amongst the people of Leeds.[58] The report also contains a useful index that begins with the schedule of the streets, lanes and alleys where cases of cholera occurred. Baker lists the number of cases, male and female, recoveries and deaths. 1,817 in all, with 702 deaths. The associations being explored, as Beresford suggests, were related to the unsanitary streets rather than any link between the disease and the victims' age, sex, occupation, diet or even moral character.[59] Others were less sure, however, and the *Leeds Mercury* was eager to show that morality was one of the preservers of health and that the drunkard should 'instantly make his will'.[60]

The initial thinking, and indeed reporting, inclined towards the view that the disease only attacked the lowest classes in society. Reports indicated that the victims were usually poor and 'living in a depraved and immoral manner'.[61] In late 1831 Samuel Smith, 'one of the best known and most respected of Leeds surgeons,'[62] and William Hey, the Tory Mayor of Leeds and also a surgeon, who was elected surgeon to the infirmary on the retirement of his father William,[63] visited the North East. When they returned they reported that only three 'respectable people' had been attacked in Newcastle. The rest appeared to be either addicted to alcohol or living in crowded apartments. This view was also implied in a report from that area that appeared in the *Lancet*. At Newburn, 'a place of trifling extent', some five miles from Newcastle, readers were informed that the rector 'and other persons of comparative opulence fell its ready victims'.[64]

It is true, of course, as Baker points out that the victims tended to come from the poorer areas of Leeds. His report shows that in the areas that had been drained, paved and sewered and cleansed there were 245 cases of cholera. However, in the other half of the town where an equal number of people lived where there was neither street cleansing nor sewers, 1203 cases occurred.[65]

The papers were slow to point out that not all the victims were from the poorer areas of the town, although the death of the sister-in-law of the editor of the *Yorkshire Gazette* may have changed their views.[66] Some of the business and professional people would begin to realise this when reports such as the one, for example, from the *Leeds Mercury* in August indicated that, 'several persons in respectable and comfortable positions have been attacked'.[67] Clearly it was now becoming obvious that although the majority of victims came from the poorer areas of the town, one thing was certain, cholera respected neither age, beauty nor wealth. The sudden onset of the disease, wrote Fraser Brockington, filled the hearts of the high and low alike with awe.[68]

The better off people did not appear, however, to have fled the town to the nearby spa towns of Harrogate or Ilkley. They must have been tempted, though, when they read that Harrogate had never had what was described as a more bustling season and was full of the 'best company'. Its entire freedom from cholera made it doubly desirable as a 'summer lounge.'[69] This action contrasts sharply with the views of James Kay when writing about the Manchester epidemic. He believed that the wealthier people there saw the poorer people as a threat of disease.[70]

Burying the Dead, Trying to Save the Living

The epidemic raged throughout the summer months and reached its zenith in August 1832. The scale of human suffering during that month is clear from the evidence contained in the burial register of Leeds Parish Church (St Peter's) and the adjacent daughter church of St Mary. During August alone there were 368 burials in the churchyards and 241 were of cholera victims. On the twenty-first day of that month the curate James L. Brown, buried twenty people, nineteen at St Mary's. Ten of the victims had died in hospital. On the following day a further ten were buried, eight of whom were cholera victims. The eldest was aged 72, the second eldest 36 and the youngest three weeks. Brown and John Urquhart, who was, it is believed, also a curate and who added clerk after his name (for clerk in holy orders), appear to have been responsible for most of the burials although Richard Fawcett was the vicar. Occasionally the name of J. W. Whiteley, who added officiating minister after his signature, appears in the register. He was, perhaps, another curate or a locum from another parish. All three men mentioned above helpfully wrote 'cholera', when applicable, in the right hand margin, in addition to the usual information related to abode, age and such.[71]

The first death from the disease to be recorded in the parish register, on 29 May, is that of John Dock of Bank, who is listed as an Irish cholera victim. The Irish prefix continued for two more deaths and was then dropped. A second death, again a resident of Bank, is recorded on 31 May. The aforementioned Boot and Shoe Yard makes its first appearance in the register in relation to the epidemic on 7 June when four people from that address were buried. Martha Taylor aged seventy was one of the victims, as was her husband twenty-four hours later. He was a widower for but a day. The final victim of the epidemic recorded in the register is Michael Wilson, aged forty-six, of Bridge Street who was buried on 26 December by the over worked James Brown.

How glad he must have been when the epidemic was over, and even the year, as there had been a total of 1867 burials in the parish during the past twelve months, an average of thirty-five a week.[72] Between May and November the clergy buried 1,395 people, an increase from the same period during 1831 of 415.[73] During the whole of 1832, 546 cholera victims were buried in the two churchyards. This suggests, of course, that perhaps around a hundred or so of the cholera victims

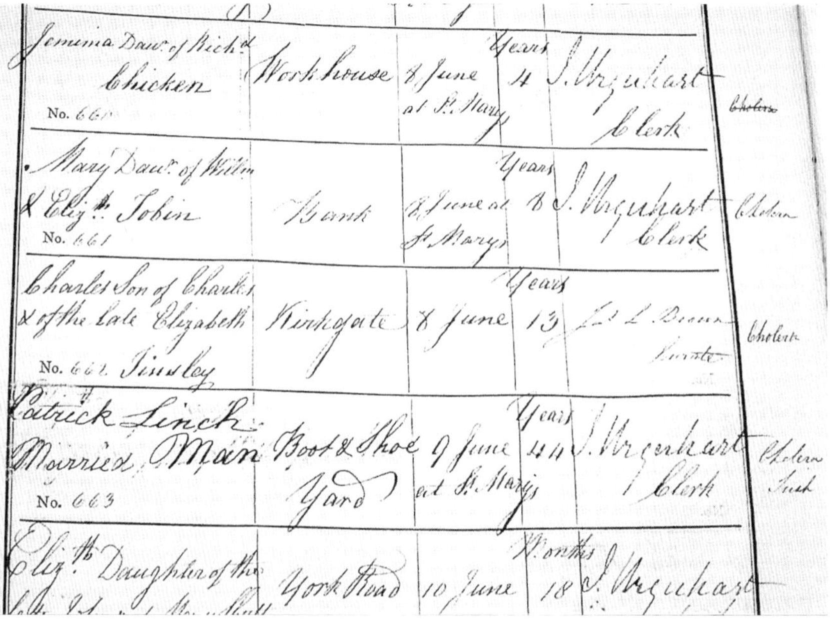

Jemima Daur. of Richd. Chicken No. 660	Workhouse	8 June at St. Mary	4 Years	J. Urquhart Clerk	Cholera
Mary Daur. of Willm. & Elizth. Tobin No. 661	Bank	8 June at St. Mary	8 Years	J. Urquhart Clerk	Cholera
Charles Son of Charles & of the late Elizabeth Tinsley No. 662	Kirkgate	8 June	13 Years	Jas. L. Brown Curate	Cholera
Patrick Linch Married Man No. 663	Boot & Shoe Yard	9 June at St. Mary	44 Years	J. Urquhart Clerk	Cholera Irish
Elizth. Daughter of the [illegible]	York Road	10 June	18 Months	J. Urquhart	

Figure 3:6 St. Peter's burial register. Detail from June 1832.
(West Yorkshire Archive Service, Leeds, Ref: RDP68/3B/7)
The five victims shown here all lived in the notoriously bad south eastern area of the town.

would have died from other causes irrespective of the epidemic. It is also interesting to note that there were 144 fewer baptisms than the previous three years' average recorded in the registers during 1832. The victims' stated abodes also cover very many of the streets listed by Robert Baker. The highest percentage, eleven per cent, came from Bank an area that included a number of folds including the Boot and Shoe Yard. Although fifty-four patients died in hospital, on only two occasions is the *cholera* hospital specifically recorded in the register as the patients' abode at the time of their death. The victims named are James Kay, aged twelve, and David Whindle, forty-five.

However, as the records show, the high rate of infant mortality in the town ensured that both James Brown and John Urquhart were burying people on a regular basis irrespective of the cholera epidemic. On 8 April, for example, before the epidemic began, the former had buried eight parishioners six of whom were aged three and under.[74] It is not surprising that by 1842 these burial grounds were over full and, in the case of the Parish Church, in 'a disgusting state', and the Beckett Street cemetery, at Burmantofts, was opened by the town council in 1845.[75] This was to prove a wise decision, for when cholera returned to the town with a vengeance in 1849, between forty and fifty people were being buried there daily 'in all weathers' between 8am and midnight, by three clergymen.[76]

During the height of the epidemic the Board had had little success in containing the spread of the disease and the many cures suggested by both the medical profession and others, had no effect. The mortality rate from the disease during the 1832 epidemic was around 35 per cent and Robert Baker also provides us, in the

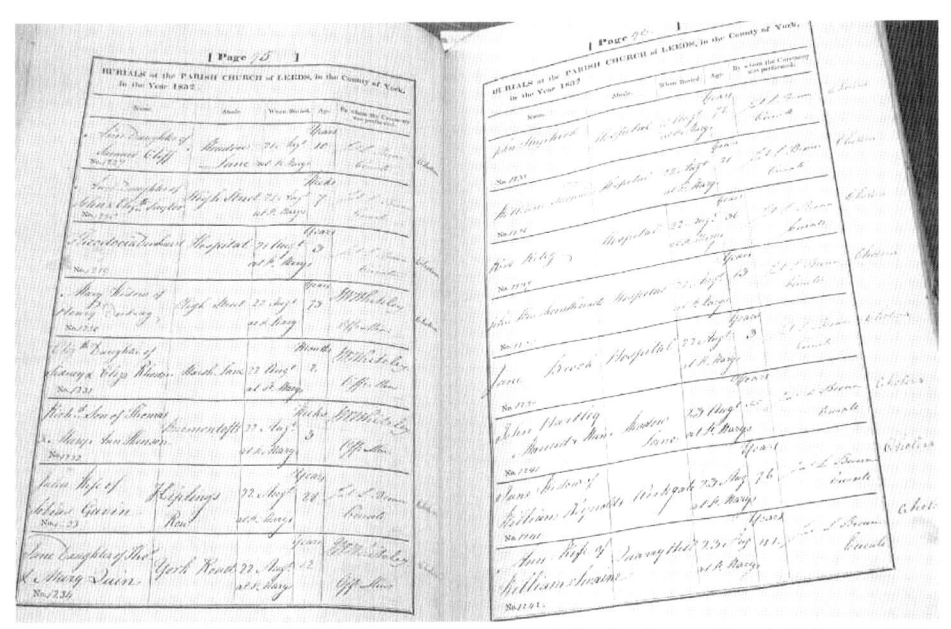

Figure 3:7 St. Peter's burial register, showing sixteen of the deaths on 24 and 25 August 1832.
(West Yorkshire Archive Service, Leeds. Ref: RDP68/3B/7)
Thirteen people are recorded here as victims of the epidemic, by the clergy. The other three burials are all of children under one year.[77]

appendix to his report, with details of the age and sex distribution of the cases under what Underwood describes as 'the curious title' of 'A Calculation on the Probabilities of Human existence in Persons attacked by Cholera, in every age, from six months to ninety years, both inclusive'. Underwood helpfully provides the reader with an abbreviated statement, as shown below.[78]

Table 3:1 Age and sex distribution of mortality. Leeds, 1832

Age	-5	-10	-20	-30	-40	-50	-60	-70	70+	Age Unknown	Total
Cases	151	139	193	215	307	310	179	125	77	121	1817
Deaths	76	45	51	60	89	104	100	80	56	41	702
Case mortality %	50	32	27	28	29	34	56	64	73	-	38.7%

From this it is clear that the disease was extremely fatal during the early years of life and that the case mortality rate increased again from around the age of fifty. The gender survival rate can also be ascertained form Baker's report. 971 females contracted the disease and 362 (37.2 per cent died). This was a slighty better figure than the death rate of 40 per cent (340 in number) amongst the 846 males who were inflicted. The disease, of course, had no known cure, and how the victims must have suffered when many of the 'remedies' were administered. Many, in fact, must have done more harm than good. It is still frustrating to read that even the practice of injecting saline fluid into the clearly dehydrated patients was deemed by Baker to be of little success and was not continued.[79]

Cruel Lives

In a letter to the *Lancet* Dr. Richard Birtwhistle supports this view, when he 'regrets to state' that it (Saline injection) had not been found to answer the sanguine expectations that its first announcement created. Mr. Teale, the surgeon of the Holbeck cholera hospital, did not think himself justified in again 'having recourse' to it unless it proved to be more successful. When a patient was admitted to the hospital in a collapsed state, attempts were made to restore natural temperature with suitably shaped hot water tins. Additional stimulants of ammonia and camphor were administered. A 'scruple of calomel' was then given every hour until the symptoms eased. In addition to the oral remedies tried there was often the added discomfort of enemas. The latter were administered at the hospital in Marsh Lane, Leeds by Mr. Morley the resident surgeon who, however, had not had sufficient experience to enable him to form an opinion of their value! At nearby York, patients received enemas of spirits of turpentine in some 'thick mucilaginous' medium. This, apparently, restrained the 'excessive and exhausting evacuations' and was deemed to be worthy of a more extensive trial.[80]

Charles Thackrah, a founder member of the Leeds School of Medicine that opened in October, 1831,[81] offers a variety of options in his seminal work, published in Leeds in 1832, on the treatment of cholera. The treatment he stresses must be 'founded on a correct view of the nature of the malady, and have close regard to stage and circumstance'. Stimulants were required but their employment had to be administered with reference to the state of the blood. If this was so thick as to impair the action of the heart and blood vessels then bleeding was recommended. This is one of the many options advocated for use 'in particular circumstances' and the options are classified according to the stages at which they should be administered. His final rallying cry to his colleagues is that:

Apathy, fear and despair, are as great evils in the practitioner, as a sinking circulation in the patient. [82]

Thackrah's contribution to medical science was considered by the first Chief Medical Officer, John Simon, to be comparable with that of Edward Jenner. Thackrah did not, however, live to see all of his work bear fruition as he died of tuberculosis in 1833, aged 38.[83] In addition to the 'cures' being used there was much advice with regard to prevention. This began as early as June when the Board advised that 'all filth and wet should be carefully removed from the house'. Further suggestions included the need to avoid intemperance, to use 'garden stuff' sparingly and to abstain from 'luscious meat'. Most of this advice was achievable but it is difficult to see how many in the town could follow the guidance to 'wash whole person with soap and water at least once a week'.[84]

Local companies were quick to advertise their preventative wares. Typical of many advertisements is one for 'Mr. Baker's Improved Foot and Body Warmers' available from T. Turkington and Company in Briggate. They were eager to 'by leave and most respectfully' inform medical gentlemen of Leeds that these had been found to be most effectual in cases of cholera, colds, rheumatism and inflammatory diseases.[85] When it came to cholera and bowel complaints in general, readers of the *Intelligencer* were advised by Dicey and Company to obtain their genuine 'Daffy's

Elixir' at two shillings or two shillings and nine pence a bottle (approximately, perhaps, a quarter of what most of the victims would be earning each week) and to ensure that they took care to ask the chemist only for 'Dicey's Daffy' and to check that the company's name was stamped on the bottle.[86]

Letters from medical men appeared in the papers on a regular basis. Each seemed to have his personal special cure or preventative potion, and was eager to pass the information on to the public. Mr. Felton, a surgeon from Liverpool, was of the 'firm belief' that carbonate of soda and ginger-twenty grams of the former and eight grams of the latter- taken three times a week after morning and evening meals in a wine glass of water, will act as an effective prevention.[87] The 'eminent surgeon', Mr. Hope, recommended an ounce of peppermint water and camphor mixture with forty drops of tincture of opium, a fourth part of which was to be served in a portion of gruel every three of four hours.[88] Francis Sharpe, a local house surgeon, had devised a lightweight hot air system based on the one used in hospital, which could be used under the bedclothes.[89] In similar vein a letter from one who signed himself 'Theta' recommended a spirit hot air bath that could be obtained from most respectable ironmongers in Leeds.[90]

It is difficult to know just how many of these preventative methods and cures were obtained, but however genuine the reasons for the letters were, they do, now, appear to be extremely misguided. How many people, one wonders, tried the following dubious remedy published in the *Intelligencer* and recalled by Smith?

Two large spoonfuls of tincture of rhubarb, twelve drops of sal volatile and five drops of the essence of peppermint mixed together with a wine glass full of hot water.

If the patient was not much better after this apparent elixir of life, the whole process could be repeated in an hour.[91]

The *Leeds Mercury's* editor Edward Baines, who had turned the paper into 'the most influential provincial paper in the country'[92] was eager to stress as early as October, 1831 that places such as Kirkgate that were 'nests of vice and filth and receptacles of everything that is infamous' ought to be cleared out as they were 'hot beds of infection'. Baines, was a powerful man, who was described by Engels as a bourgeois economist and publicist.[93] The paper was also eager to stress that intemperance had much to answer for and that temperance and morality were the only preservatives of health.[94]

The Board, as we would expect, also published a list of preventative measures and some of these have already been alluded to. The three key elements being general and personal cleanliness, regular and frequent ventilation, along with the whitewashing of apartments. Temperance, citizens were informed, was of the highest importance.[95] The latter is an interesting point as when cholera attacked the people of London in 1854 it was the anti bacterial properties of beer, and all fermented spirits, that proved to be safer than the local water supplies. For much of human history, suggests Johnson, the answer to diseases such as dysentery, was to drink alcohol.[96]

Treatment recommended by the Board included the need to wrap the patient in warm blankets until advice could be sought from a medical man. Above all, there was the need for 'calmness of mind and fortitude' and the hope that 'under the blessing of Divine providence', what appeared to be almost the inevitable approach of the disease could be prevented and its progress arrested.[97] Many did turn to God both immediately before, and during the epidemic. During the years preceding the epidemic there had been a decline in church attendance and two thirds of the people of Leeds had never been to a service.[98] A reliance on the protection and providence of God would, wrote Thackrah, enable the people to 'meet with resolution the evils of life and often saves us from the worst'.[99] The government supported this view with a national day of fasting, humiliation and prayer on 21 March 1832. In Leeds all but a few shops were closed, workers had a day of rest and the population conducted themselves in a solemn manner.[100] There were those who thought that the epidemic was a call to prayer and a Leeds milliner Robert Ayrey wrote to his brother suggesting that religion in Leeds was in a 'state of lukewarmness' and 'this plague' was a call to stir people up.[101]

A 'Disgusting Trade'

The epidemic did stir people up but not in the way that Ayrey predicted. There was a belief in the town, particularly amongst the poorer classes, that cholera was a result of a plot between the doctors and the wealthier classes to do away with the poor. This misguided view amongst the lower classes of Leeds was based on a general suspicion of the doctors linked to the schools of anatomy, the general fear of and unknown nature of the disease, and the recent Reform Bill.[102] The latter had given more power to the people following the redistribution of parliamentary seats. Leeds, previously unrepresented, was to have two members of parliament. Although the trouble in Leeds, the stoning of the hospital, the withdrawal of patients and the violence, had grown from seeds sown over a period of time, it was the raging epidemic that showed little sign of abating that acted as a propagator.

The Leeds Anatomy School had been established in 1831 and appears to have relied initially on an agreement with the Leeds Workhouse Board that bodies of poor persons who died in the workhouse and were unclaimed by relatives should be given for dissection.[103] Other less desirable practices were also responsible for a supply of bodies to the school of anatomy and these were continuing.

One of the incidents that was reported in the *Leeds Mercury* long before the cholera outbreak, and may almost have gone unnoticed by the majority of those in the town, clearly involved Robert Baker although he was never charged. During the weekend of 11-12 March, 1826 the body of 15 year old Martha Oddy, who died after a very short illness, was removed from the Chapel Yard at Armley, a few miles from the centre of Leeds. On the following Monday it was noticed that the grave was open, the body gone and only the clothes left behind. Three men were quickly apprehended. Following questioning, two of the men were released and only Thomas Smith detained. It quickly emerged that a key culprit was a Michael

Armstrong, who was not one of the three arrested initially. He was located at a lodging house in Doncaster and brought back to Leeds 'heavily ironed'. He allegedly had been persuaded by Smith to remove the body.

When the pair were before magistrates on the following Friday, it emerged that the 'most material evidence as affecting Armstrong' was that given by one Robert Baker. He acknowledged that he had seen Armstrong, initially three months earlier, and had met him for a second time on the previous Monday, at five in the morning following a message from a friend. When they met Armstrong, and another man whom Baker did not know, had a sack with them containing the body of a female. The witness (Baker) we are told gave Armstrong four pounds for the body and took it away. It was in his possession until Tuesday night when he left it at 'the cross roads'. He did this, he indicated, so that 'the friends of the deceased ' could recover it! Other witnesses said that as soon as Baker saw the placards indicating that the body was missing he 'became desirous that it should be returned'. If he had wanted to conceal his involvement in the transaction he had, he suggested, had sufficient time to dispose of the body.

The outcome of the case was that Armstrong was bailed to appear at the next sessions and Smith was remanded for further examination. Baker simply left the court along with other witnesses. Martha Oddy was re-interred at Armley shortly

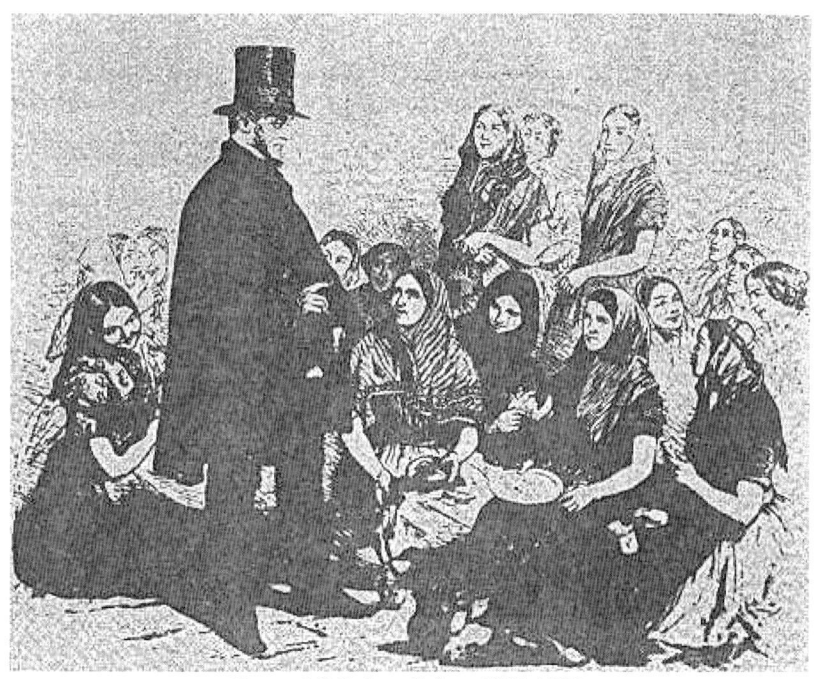

Figure 3:8 Robert Baker, 1803-1880.
(British Journal of Industrial Medicine. Volume 21, 1964)

Baker is seen here with Yorkshire factory girls. His 1833 report in relation to the Leeds cholera epidemic, and a follow up report in 1839, were described many years later, by the chairman of the Royal Sanitary Commission, to be 'greatly in advance of what had been done up to that time in such matters'[104] afterwards at 'a very early hour'. The paper makes no comment whatsoever other than to condemn the practice of body snatching. There is, however, a final extremely interesting and telling paragraph that is again reported without any comment. We read that the body, when found, was in a box 'only' two feet in length, fourteen inches in breadth and ten inches in depth. It was coiled in it with so much skill that not a bone was broken.[105]

Six years later at the beginning of the epidemic, on 5 April 1832, the *Leeds Intelligencer* had reported the case of a partial exhumation of a body at Oulton, a community six miles to the south east of the town centre. 'Great excitement was occasioned', readers were informed, by the circumstances relating to the body and grave of John Hutchins. The grave, when checked, had presented a spectacle that was 'truly revolting'. Prior to the perpetrators of this act of body snatching being disturbed, a rope had been attached to the corpse and several instruments used in what was described as a 'disgusting trade' were scattered nearby along with a bottle of rum.[106]

In the same edition of the paper there was a detailed report of a court case in relation to charge of disinterment of a body on 2 November 1831. Five young men aged between nineteen and twenty-five were accused that they did 'severally, wickedly, willingly and unlawfully, conspire, combine, cooperate and agree together' to disinter a dead body at East Ardsley, a village seven miles south of Leeds.[107] A week earlier the paper reported an incident in Scotland where an 'untenanted' coffin of a patient, whose body had been stolen, was paraded in Paisley.[108]

It was also around the time of this court case, on 11 November, that a box had arrived at the Bull and Mouth Hotel in Briggate (renamed the Grand Central in 1903 and the Victory in 1921. It was demolished to make way for Woolworth's in 1939),[109] by coach from Manchester containing the bodies of a woman and child. Addressed to a Revd. Mr. Gilleste, Hull, possibly a fictional clergyman, and marked suspiciously 'to be left until called for. Glass and keep this way up'. Anning quotes Mayhall who recorded in his annals that the Hull School had not yet started but they (the bodies) would not be carried in this way unless 'intended for dissection'[110]

It wasn't just news of body snatching that was reaching the people of Leeds. There was also news of premature burial in the national press and in February 1832 the Times reported two 'distressing cases'. One was the case of a boy who kicked the coffin lid on his way to the graveyard. The other was the case of a man who was convinced that his wife was alive and threatened to kill anyone who nailed down the coffin lid. Spasms were common symptoms in cholera victims but in these cases both were reported later to be alive.[111] In some cases it could be, suggests Durey, that inexperienced or frightened medical men had incorrectly diagnosed death, especially as there was a need for a quick burial.[112] The Leeds people would, no doubt, get to hear of these cases and emotions were soon running high.

On 14 June, the *Leeds Intelligencer* reported the case of a Mrs. Burke, 63, a resident of Blue Bell Fold who despite 'shrunken eyes, blueness, coldness, shrivelled fingers and contracted body, had refused to go into hospital. Was she, one wonders, already aware of the rumours circulating with regard to medical research?[113]

Suspicions, Fears and Civil Unrest

When a cholera hospital was established against the wishes of the local people, and businesses in the immediate vicinity, adjacent to St Peter's Square things began to hot up. The building had previously been used as a 'lying in' hospital and was to have the 'well respected ' figure of George Morley, who had run a similar institution in London, as its house surgeon.[114] Suspicion was quickly cast on the activities of the doctors whom, it was thought, wanted to use the hospital for their own purposes.[115] It wasn't just the fear that bodies were being used for anatomical research. Rumours were now also coming from Europe that cholera was a 'Malthusian plot' between the doctors and the middle classes, as we have heard, to kill the poor off by luring them to the hospital that would become something of a human abattoir.[116]

All cases of fever in Leeds, whatever the nature, had since November 1804 been sent to the somewhat optimistically named House of Recovery in Vicar Lane. A location uncomfortably close, notes Barnard, to the most unhealthy area of the town.[117] All persons 'labouring under infectious fever and unable to provide either medicines or proper accommodation' were admissible. Although temporary additional buildings were added, it became too small to cope with the epidemic and additional and more specialist provision had to be provided.[118]

On 9 June an angry crowd surrounded the cholera hospital building, threw stones and broke many windows. They remained all weekend and the atmosphere remained tense. However, after the initial flurry of stones, the crowds that collected around the square were content to express their angry feelings by offensive shouting and threats'. The following week the *Intelligencer* made the understated pronouncement that:

Considerable dissatisfaction has been manifested by the inhabitants, and owners, of property in St Peter's Square, at the cholera hospital being appointed in that area. [119]

The case of Margaret Leeson appeared to be the catalyst of much of the trouble after what was initially described as 'passive opposition' by the crowd. On 9 June Mrs. Leeson, who had arrived in Leeds recently from Hull, was apparently attacked with cholera in the notorious Boot and Shoe Yard, where she had stayed the previous evening. She was admitted to hospital and appeared to 'be happy'. However, when her husband left the hospital after accompanying her he was confronted by what is described as an 'excitable group' and persuaded, following their suspicions that she was to be murdered, to remove his wife. When he re-entered the hospital to do just that he was, in turn, met by George Morley, the surgeon. He was then happy to accept Morley's explanation and left without his wife.

However, the poor man must have been thrown into a further state of confusion and distress when, on reaching the street, he was once more confronted by the small crowd. Again he was encouraged to re-enter the hospital to remove his wife, now with promises that they, the protestors, would look after her. This he did but whilst he was remonstrating with the staff Mrs. Leeson leapt out of a window!

The patient, readers were informed, could be seen at 17 Boot and Shoe Yard. There is no record, however, of how many people, if any, chose to visit this site.[120] A site, it is worth repeating, that was being described in the *Leeds Mercury* published the morning of the day of the incident, as a 'receptacle of poverty, misery and uncleanliness' and that there were few places in the town more likely to generate disease as this.[121]

Her escape from hospital did little to calm the angry mob that continued, we read, to lurk outside the hospital. 'Vollies (sic) of stones' began to fly and several windows were smashed. During the night several people, described as ruffians, approached the building as 'if by concert' to make further attacks. The angry group remained on the following day and continued to shout and threaten those in authority but no more stones were thrown.[122]

On the same day a billposter, William Thomas, was apprehended by a police constable while posting bills that clearly inflamed the situation. The bills carried the bold headline, 'Cholera Morbus Hunters Taken in Trap'. The bills, or posters, that ridiculed the doctors appeared all over the town. They reported that people were convinced that Margaret Leeson was drunk and did not have cholera. She had been rescued from 'premature death', by being removed from the hospital. Her husband, it was claimed, had been unable to visit this wife and, it was rumoured, the surgeon had been eager to retain his 'pretended patient'. Suspicion was further cast on the doctors' motives when it was learned that patients were not allowed to leave the hospital of their own free will, nor was anybody allowed to pay their last respects to friends and relatives who had died in the hospital. Thomas was fined £5, say more than five weeks' wages, and 7s 4d (37p) costs for posting the bills 'without the printer's name'. He was later sent to the house of correction in Wakefield as he failed to pay the fine.[123]

Smith suggests that the posters were the work of local manufacturers who resented the presence of the hospital on their door-step. They were unashamedly using fears of the working class, to put pressure on the Board of Health to move the hospital. The manufacturers also feared that quarantine regulations being enforced would affect their businesses especially as those who were exporting had to issue certificates to prove that the area was free from cholera. The way the disease was communicated was, of course, little understood, but given the fears that it could be passed on through manufactured commodities, it is fair to say that the hospital would not have been good for business.[124]

The Board of health did take note of the concerns expressed in relation to the hospital's location. Having 'looked again' at the situation a new site at Saxton Lane, a quarter of a mile to the east of the town, was purchased within days for

£550. A committee was formed in relation to the establishment of the hospital there, and work began immediately. Whilst the new hospital was being prepared the St Peter's site remained open for those who wanted to use it. However, this may have satisfied the business people but others were clearly less easy to satisfy. When the news spread, again an angry crowd of both sexes gathered and there was more verbal abuse. A member of the newly formed committee, Mr. S. Smith, was physically attacked when leaving the site in Saxton Lane. The offender, one Patrick Burke, was arrested and fined five pounds. As in the case of the billposter, he was unable to pay and sent to the house of correction for two months.[125]

The hospital remained open until 22 November when the Board made the decision to close it. The town was pronounced officially free from the disease on 23 November although a few fatalities did occur after this date. As we have seen the last known victim, according to the burial register, was one Michael Wilson who was buried 26 December 1832.[126]

By the end of the year the pestilence had caused 1,960 deaths in the county. In addition to the 702 deaths in Leeds, 402 died in Sheffield, 300 in Hull, 185 in York and sixty-two in Wakefield. Bradford, so close to Leeds, had fewer than forty deaths.[127] Across Britain the disease killed roughly 32,000 people during late 1831, and 1832. Three other epidemics in 1849, 1854 and 1866 (the final one) were, in turn, responsible for 62,000, 20,000 and 14,000 deaths nationwide.[128]

Epilogue

When the epidemic was over life for the people of Leeds continued very much as before. It was as though the cholera had never visited the town, as the epidemic did not produce any immediate commitment to public health.[129]

Robert Baker presented his report to the Leeds Board of Health on 21 January 1833. It left members in no doubt about the task facing them. The appalling conditions in which people were living was clear from the text. Additionally, Baker added statistics and cartography to the appendix. There were a few cosmetic measures carried out such as the whitewashing of the Boot and Shoe Yard at, it was reported, 'public expense'! This cosmetic ritual, as Beresford puts it, was, however, surpassed at the equally notorious Blue Bell Fold. It merely had its name removed from the street maps and directories, and was rechristened. A reference to 'Tindall's Yard, otherwise called Blue Bell Yard', appears in old deeds but there is no mention of the original name in the 1841 census.[130] Baker was, suggests Sylvia Barnard, 'a prophet crying in the wilderness'.[131] His report of 1842 to Edwin Chadwick still paints a dreadful picture of the town and could almost have been written ten years earlier at the height of the epidemic. In fact in an interim 1839 report Baker noted that, for example, excrement was still an issue in the Blue Bell Fold and that it had not been removed since the 1832 clearance.[132]

Chadwick was fascinated with the prospect of Baker also coming forward with a 'Sanatory (sic) Map' of Leeds and illustrating, with the aid of this, the correlation between disease and housing.[134] The River Aire, said Baker, was still 'discoloured'

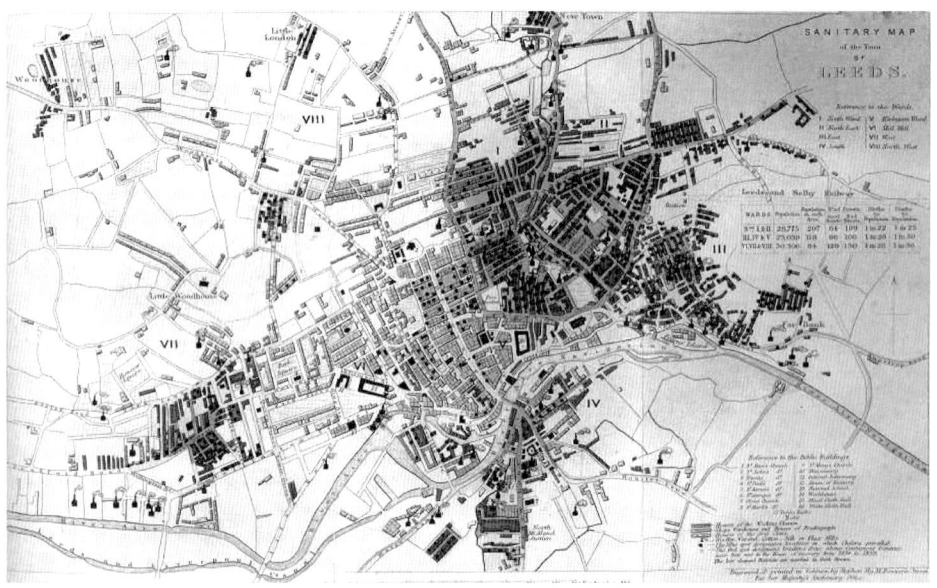

Figure 3:9 Sanitary Map of the Town of Leeds, 1839
(Thackray Medical Museum)

Based on his original cholera plan of 1833, this 'Sanitary Map of the Town of Leeds', drawn in 1839 for an interim second report to the Leeds Board of Health, was submitted to Edwin Chadwick for his 1842 report. The spots indicate localities in which cholera prevailed and the 'less cleansed' districts are shown by dark shading.[133]

and the Timble Beck, which flowed through the most populated ward, was 'so exhalant and noisome as to be offensive in the first degree'.[135] Clearly little had changed. The 1842 Leeds Improvement Act had given the corporation powers to ease the public health problems in the town, and prohibited the occupation of houses in courtyards narrower than thirty feet.[136] It took, in fact, a further and more intense cholera epidemic, in 1849, to stimulate some action.[137] Real progress was, however, only made following the Leeds Improvement Act of 1866 and even this failed to prohibit back-to-back houses.[138]

When the appalling conditions that many of the people of Leeds were living in, and continued to do so, were coupled with the high mortality rate amongst those very people it is surprising that there was not more civil unrest in 1832. The riots had been brief, and although they resulted in some modifications in relation to hospital provision in the town, they really appear to have had little long-term effect locally. As Burrell and Gill point out they were not really 'anti government' and were directed mainly at the medical profession.[139] This was very much the case in Leeds, although there is a suggestion from Morris that the people also mistrusted the 'traditional ruling agencies' of the town. Seventeen of the fifty-six members of the Board of Health had come from a previously un-elected body whose political and religious views had already been challenged.[140]

As early as November 1831, a report in the *Intelligencer* indicated that there was a feeling the board was indifferent to the plight of the majority. The feeling could have been exacerbated by the inclusion of some of the wealthy industrialists in the town. The paper named six of them. These were the same people, it went on to say, who appeared to have no hesitation when it suited them to keep wages low or to throw men out of work.[141] Clearly there was a seed for future unrest here.

When compared with the events in some other northern towns and cities, the Leeds riots were of a modest nature. Why was this? Was it that the people were worn down by the constant struggle against disease and life in general or was the answer, as Briggs implies, slightly more obtuse? The people of Leeds were fortunate, he believes, in their doctors. He cites especially Baker and Thackrah, and this may have helped to maintain an air of calmness. He also believes that in Leeds the propensity to riot was less marked than in other places such as Manchester and Bradford.[142]

This is an amended version of the author's chapter 'The Leeds Cholera Epidemic: The Pestilence Extends' in *Cholera and Conflict* Ed. M. Holland, G.Gill & S. Burrell. Published by the Medical Museum Publishing, 2009.

Chapter Four

An Aggravated Calamity

Heptonstall-Slack 1843-44: Typhus or Typhoid?

There is to hand a detailed and contemporary report by Robert Howard, surgeon, of the 1843-4 typhus epidemic entitled *History of the typhus that prevailed as an endemic in Heptonstall-Slack during the winter of 1843-4*. It is accompanied by remarks on the 'sanatory (sic) state of the village' that are directly related to the 'aggravated calamity that intruded itself' on Howard's mind.[1] The report forms the basis of this chapter in which, following an introduction to typhus and a look at a Leeds epidemic, we consider whether in fact the outbreak recorded by Howard was indeed caused by the typhus microbe.

Throughout the first half of the nineteenth century typhoid and typhus were confused with one another as their symptoms were similar; confused, in fact, to such an extent that until 1869, when they were first differentiated, they were grouped together as typhoid in the nosologies. In the first year the figures were separated there were 4,281 typhus deaths in England and Wales.[2]

Typhoid, as we shall see again in the final chapter, is a disease that, like cholera, is spread orally by contaminated water and, to a lesser extent, food. Typhus, however, is an acute infectious disease spread by the body louse (*pediculus humanus corporis*) or, to be precise, their infected faeces. The lice live and lay their eggs in the clothing of humans and then, after nipping the blood of an infected person, move to another person. They now leave infected excrement that is easily rubbed into the blood stream by scratching. The causative agent was named *Rickettsial prowazeki* after the two scientists* who substantiated the previous research carried out at the beginning of the twentieth century.[3] It is an environmental disease that can only survive where there is a lack of personal and household cleanliness. After an incubation period of anything from a week to fourteen days there is a high fever, severe head, muscle and joint aches and eventually a characteristic dark rash caused by bleeding into the skin. In most cases the microbe invades the brain causing delirium, seizures and stupor.[4]

The spread of the disease was greatly encouraged by overcrowded properties, and the many names by which it was known reinforce this point. For example, gaol fever, ship fever, hunger fever and camp fever. The workhouse proved to be an

---

* Howard Taylor Ricketts (1871-1910) and Stanislaus von Prowazeki (1875-1915). Both died from a fatal dose of typhus whilst trying to identify its causes. [5]

attractive breeding ground for the microbe. The mortality rate was high and often as many as one third of cases ended in death. It was immortalised, Anne Hardy reminds us, by Charles Dickens in *Bleak House*. In the slum of Tom-all-Alone's fever houses the dead and dying were carried out like 'sheep with the rot'. By the end of the nineteenth century typhus had ceased to be of significant concern, the only one of what Hardy refers to as 'the communicable diseases in the nineteenth century preventive canon' about which that could be said.[6] However, before that time the disease proved to be a major killer, with major outbreaks, especially in towns such as Leeds, throughout the land.

Typhus also had profound effects upon the fortunes of war, again when a number of people are herded together, wearing the same clothes day after day and lacking the facilities to ensure bodily cleanliness. For example, in 1812 Napoleon's army was in the fatal grip of an outbreak of typhus. A year later the army was defeated, as a 'result of typhus fever, cold, hunger' and, it is suggested, Napoleon himself who was not only in poor health but had 'sacrificed reality for a dream'.[7]

Leeds, 1847

Before we consider the outbreak in Heptonstall–Slack it may be useful to look first at Leeds in 1847. The town, as we have already seen, grew rapidly from the beginning of the nineteenth century. It had already suffered an alarming outbreak of typhus fever earlier in the century, in 1801-02,[8] and the gross overcrowding and inadequate sanitation was tested even further in early 1847. It was then, following famine in Ireland in 1846, that thousands of Irish people fled the horrors of starvation and descended on towns such as Liverpool and Leeds where many Irish families had already settled. The Bank area of Leeds was already established as 'an area of cramped houses, little in the way of sanitation, rampant ill health with an accompanying high rate of mortality', so vividly described by Helen Kennally.[9] We read that 'wretchedness, filth and disease' predominated there, especially in Goulden's Buildings (a notorious location - see figure 2:4) and Back York Street. It was to this area in south-east Leeds, then, that the Irish immigrants came in vast numbers. It was into this grossly overcrowded environment that typhus also found a ready welcome.

As summer came the population increased rapidly, especially in the Kirkgate and East Wards, where families were 'ravaged' by typhus. In the latter ward, on the Bank, it was reported that in Brighton Court there were fourteen people, including nine children, sick in two houses. Neither house had a bed. Cellar dwellings were common and in two 'homes', again without beds, in Lower Cross Street, seven people were sick with the fever.[10]

Beds were, of course, breeding grounds in themselves, especially when shared by up to six people but the alternative, with perhaps straw or rags on the floor, would be equally attractive to body lice. Kennally records that hundreds died during 1847 from the effects of starvation and fever, and 1,525 Irish burials were recorded at the Parish Church. The distress is again hard to imagine for, as we have seen during the Leeds measles outbreak, multiple deaths occurred within a single family. Mary Rape, a resident of Foundry Street lost her husband on 17 May 1847, followed

Cruel Lives

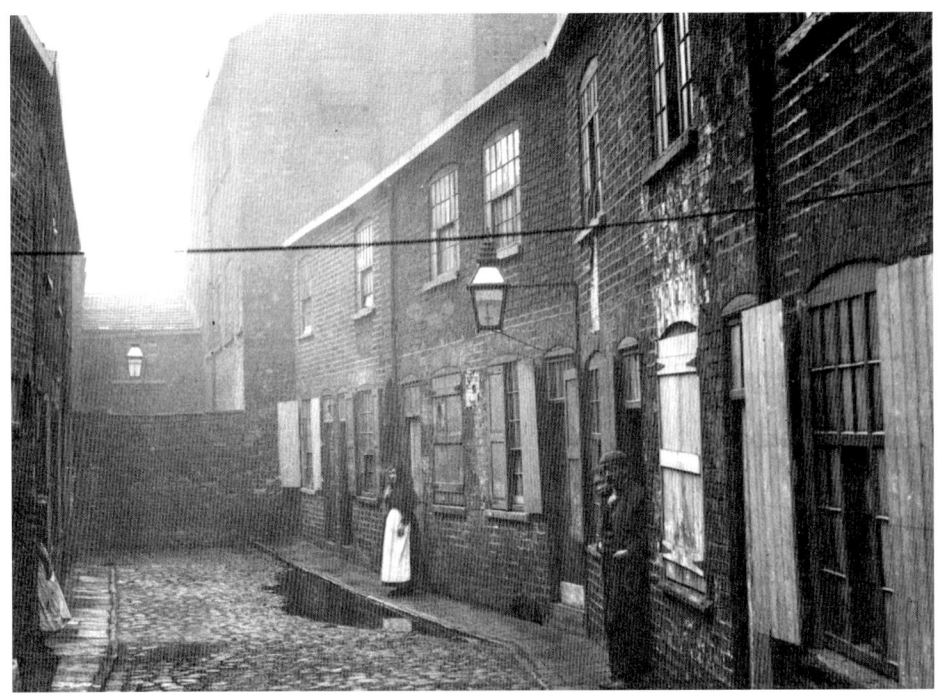

Figure 4:1 Goulden's Square off York Street.
(Leeds Library and Information Service www.leodis.net)

during the next four weeks by five of her children. Thomas and Ellen Keenan lost three children within a week at the end of October.[11]

Generally typhus found a home, as we have seen, in the cramped and unhygienic properties of the poor. It did, however, during the 1847 Leeds outbreak, attack many others such as clergy and medical people who did their best to reduce the suffering of the victims. On 1 September the death of Elizabeth Warwick, matron of the convalescent hospital, was reported. She had caught the disease when 'discharging her duties'. The outbreak also claimed the lives of five Catholic priests from St Anne's and St Patrick's.[12] All had fallen victim to what one registrar referred to as their 'indefatigable attentions to the poor of their church'.[13]

One of the saddest cases concerned a young Anglican curate from Berkshire, William Stanley Monck. His life in Leeds has been extensively and lovingly recorded by Gillian Figures. Monck was ordained deacon on 28 February 1847 just before his twenty-fifth birthday. He died from typhus less than five months later on the ninth of July. During that short time he had ministered to those in some of the worst areas of the Bank. In one cellar he reported finding 'thirty-one men, women and children all lying on the damp filthy floor'. In another cellar, which he helped to clean with a colleague, he found nineteen people suffering from typhus. In addition to such duties Monck was, like those clergymen to whom we have referred in chapter three, burying large numbers on a daily basis. On 21 March he conducted fifteen burials of which twelve were for children under the age of five. An illuminated window, now forgotten and placed in a store-room at the Parish

Church, was dedicated to his memory. Attempts are being made to restore the window and create what Gillian Figures aptly refers to as 'a fitting tribute to a young man's sacrifice'.[14]

Slack: 1843-4

What, though, are we to make of the alleged typhus outbreak in Heptonstall-Slack, near Halifax during the winter of 1843-4? The outbreak began during September 1843 and terminated around 14 February of the following year. It has, however, been included here as a fine example of the confusion that often occurred, and to ask the question: was this actually an outbreak of *typhoid* fever? There were fifty-one cases and eight deaths amongst the population of around 348 of whom 184 were twenty years of age and under and only forty-five were fifty and older. The epidemic is well documented, as already indicated, in a detailed paper by Robert Howard, a surgeon. His report, *History of the Typhus in Heptonstall-Slack* includes, as indicated, accompanying remarks related to the 'sanatory (sic) state' of the village.[15] These remarks will prove to be central to the debate and will, I suggest, provide an answer to the initial question. Howard's hope at the time of writing was that:

A copy or two of this inadequate production may survive and the perusal relieve the tedium of a winter's evening, by affording the reader, professional or otherwise, some information concerning the number of residents in the Slack, the physical condition of the working class, and the fierce malady with which they were assailed in the autumn and winter of 1843-4.[16]

Robert Howard's wish, then, that his work would survive the test of time has come true as we, some 160 years later, consider his findings.

Table 4:1 The ages of the 348 residents of Slack in 1844.[17]

Ages	Under 5	5-10	10-15	15-20	20-25	25-30	30-35	35-40	40-45	45-50	50-55	55-60	60-65	65-70	70-75	75-80
Nos.	48	59	49	37	27	16	16	23	23	14	15	11	8	6	4	1

The outbreak was, as readers will have noted, numerically small in comparison to the overwhelming majority of those that have provided the basis for this work. It did, however, have a profound effect on the small community surrounding the hamlet of Slack that is situated close to Heptonstall on the hillside above the Calder Valley.

A visitor to the community today will find it to be a popular and much sought after residential part of Calderdale. The village of Heptonstall and its neighbouring hamlet, that provides the focus for this chapter, are situated some one and half miles to the north-west of Hebden Bridge. They share a population today of around 1,200. Heptonstall is particularly well known through its close proximity to Hardcastle Crags, now owned by the National Trust, its ruined church and the present nineteenth-century one, its octagonal Methodist Church, and as the resting place, in the churchyard, of the ill-fated American poet Sylvia Plath (October, 1932-

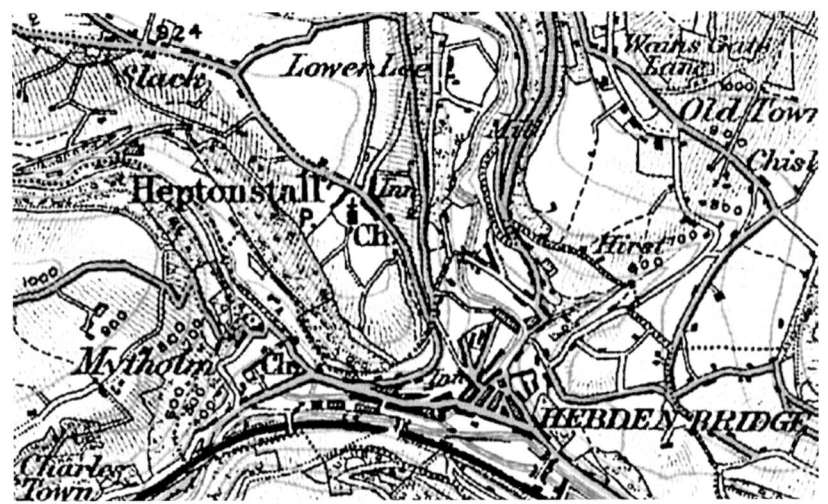

Figure 4:2 The Calder Valley c1850 showing the village of Slack in relation to Hebden Bridge and Heptonstall.
(Cassini Historical Map: Old Series, sheet 103. Original scale 1:50,000)

February, 1963). Plath, it will be recalled, was married to Ted Hughes, who was born in nearby Mytholmroyd, and was Poet Laureate from 1984 until his death in 1998.

During the time of Robert Howard, the community, chiefly consisting of hand-loom weavers, had a different feel to it when compared with today. The properties today no longer belong to those described by Howard as a class whose vocation did not require 'talent, utility or enterprise'.[18] The people wore clothes that had been 'mended and re-mended' and served for years. Many existed on a diet chiefly of oatmeal and potatoes. A typical dinner is recorded as consisting of small pieces of fried suet, with the addition of water and salt; a quantity of boiled potatoes is added, and mixed into a pulp. With this oaten bread was eaten.[19]

We can gain some understanding of life in Slack from the 1841 and 1851 census returns that precede and post date the epidemic. It is clear that life changed considerably during the 1840s due particularly to the development of the power loom that had already been introduced to, for example, Lee Mill on Hebden Water in 1832.[20] When the census enumerators visited the hamlet in 1841 they recorded that the overwhelming number of heads of households earned their living as worsted weavers. This appears to have been the case in surrounding areas, and Ian Bailey indicates that the 'dominant occupation' of heads of households in, for example, Midgley in 1841 was handloom weaving.[21] There was, however, a hint of things to come as, for example, Thomas Greenwood (the most common surname in Slack at the time), aged fourteen, is listed as power loom weaver, Thomas Haworth (50), a jobber at the factory, Betty Holt (55) a warper, and Miriam Holt (35) a reeler. However, a typical family in 1841 is still one such as John Sutcliffe, a worsted weaver, and his wife Betty, aged thirty and twenty-five respectively and their six children aged from nine years to just one. Life cannot, though, have been easy for such a family unit.

By 1851 things had begun to change profoundly and what for many, young and old, was to be a harsh life in the mills, beckoned. Houses are recorded as being unoccupied as many people moved nearer to the mills and a number of residents are listed as paupers. John Akroyd is shown as 'pauper - formerly weaver' and his wife Betty simply as 'a pauper'.[22] An indication, notes Bailey, that few hand loom weavers found employment in the mills.[23] Robert Howard, who lived in Hebden Bridge and was paid by the poor law guardians to attend to the sick, was also particularly concerned about the plight of the hand loom weavers and their loss of dignity as they had to rely on poor relief.[24]

Figure 4:3 Detail from the 1851 census return for the township of Heptonstall

Street, place or road	Name and surname	Relation to head of family	Condition	Age, male	Age, female	Occupation	Where born
Slack, north	John Akroyd*	Head	Married	67		Pauper, formerly weaver	Heptonstall
Slack, north	Betty Akroyd	Wife	Married		69	Pauper	Heptonstall

*John Akroyd is listed on the 1841 returns as a worsted weaver.

The other marked change is in the occupations listed. There is still the blacksmith, the stone-breaker and the butcher but we now also find bobbin winders, carders, and throstle spinners at the cotton mills. William Akroyd, aged forty-five, continued as a hand weaver but seven of his ten children are old enough to work, the ones aged from twenty down to nine, are each recorded as 'goes to factory-cotton'. Perhaps the mill was at Lumb Bank to the south, in the Colden Valley, where a steam engine and water wheel had been introduced at the lower mill by 1837, or one of the mills at Blackshaw Head.[25]

Throughout his remarkable report Howard makes reference to open sewers and wretched cottages that are crowded, cold, damp and dreary. The water supply came initially from three springs that fed two streams. At its origin the water from one spring situated at The Knoll was 'capital' but during the summer, as it flowed from there, it was converted into a 'nursery of loathsome animal life' that included offal from a slaughter-house. He talks also of the well, one of the many in and around Slack marked on the map (see figure 4:5), with its 'portion of human excrement' from its 'abominable contiguity' to a privy. Until the privy is demolished, he indicates, 'the water can scarcely be deemed to be fit for human uses'. It is already clear, then, that the supply of drinking water was tainted.

The focus of Howard's work then turns to the sewers and privies. It appears that the majority of the privies drained, or were situated, over cess-pools, fed by streams. The flow from the Bulyon (one of the springs) is described as follows:

The water discharges itself into a sewer: it is an open one; and previous to reaching the cottages before alluded to, [the wretched ones at the bottom of Slack] *runs through the cess pool of a privy, driving before it the agglomeration of human excrement. On its arrival at the cottages it meets another open sewer, the declination of which is from the opposite extremity of the cottages. They now unite in front of these habitations, and the commingled filth and detritus then pass through a sewer under one of the dwellings - the flags of the floor being its only covering - and the effluvi that permeates the seams is occasionally suffocative to the inmates. The refuse now makes its exit behind the house and reaccumulates in a hole prepared for its reception.*[26]

The arrangement of the privies is described in graphic detail. Around twenty-seven were provided for the 'productive class'. They were composed of rough stones, 'destitute of doors' and the only seat they possessed is described as a 'rude pole'. In front of the cesspool to these 'Temples of Cloacina' (the Roman Goddess who presided over the sewers in Roman mythology) males, females and children 'resorted' and the influence upon the morals of the population was of a 'melancholy character'.

Despite the detailed description of the water supply in the area it is not surprising to read again, as we did in chapter three, that Howard like others before him, indicates that the typhus is the result of the poisonous and noxious vapour that he found to be floating in the atmosphere. He records on a number of occasions that, for example, when one sewer was opened the exhalations overwhelmed the bystanders and resulted in nausea, vertigo and sickness. The notion of contagion was dismissed and body louse or water borne infection never even considered.

We know that the first case, during the outbreak in Slack, occurred in the home of a poor family in the centre of the village. It was a mild case and the sixteen year-

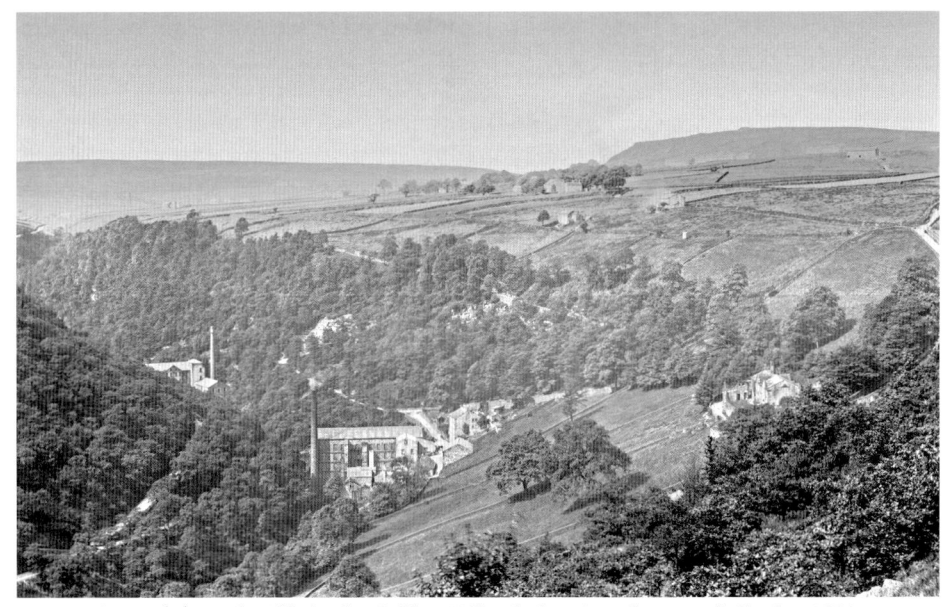

Figure 4:4 Lumb Mills in the Colden Valley below (south-west of) Slack. c1900.
(The Jack Uttley Photo Library)

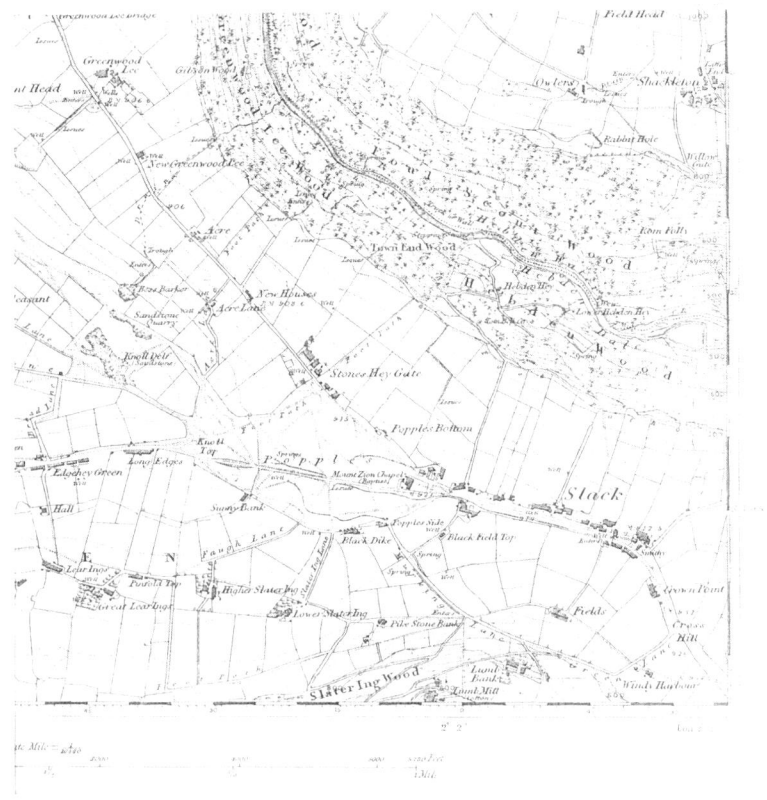

Figure 4:5 Slack Village 1848
(1:10,560 scale 1851 Ordnance Survey map)
The village of Heptonstall is just off the map, to the south-west of Slack

old male made a full recovery. Beyond that we have little information with regard to the way the disease spread and where it struck. Mention is, however, made in Howard's study of the relationship between the victims' homes and the sewers adjacent to a hole where refuse from the sewers accumulated. Three cases of fever occurred in one such house and next door there were four cases and one death. A house next to what is described as a 'covered sewer with no outlet' was home to six people who were attacked with the microbe, three of whom died.[27] However, we have no indication as to who was affected and/or died. Comparisons between the 1841 and 1851 census returns give little in the way of clues as many families had moved away during that period.

The report details some of the cases that the doctor came across and the symptoms that he witnessed. He talks of patients exhibiting a variety of symptoms and these always included in the 'well marked' cases delirium and rambling talk. In the early stages he experienced amongst other things fever, a weak pulse, accelerated respiration, 'paroxysms' of coughing sputa, or in some cases 'copious expectoration', in what appear to be a variety of unpleasant shades. In the latter stages swelling of the abdomen was a common occurrence accompanied from by, from the beginning of the fever, diarrhoea. This is described in frightening detail

Cruel Lives

Table 4:2 The ages and numbers of fever cases.

	Fever Cases Males	Females	Deaths Males	Females
Under 5 years	2	5	2	0
From 5-10	9	6	0	1
" 10-20	11	4	2	0
" 20-30	2	2	1	0
" 30-40	4	3	0	1
" 40-50	0	3	0	1
Totals	28	23	5	3

Proportion of sick to population is approximately 1: 7 and deaths to cases approximately 1: 6.5 [28]

and the description includes the fact that in certain cases the victim would pass eight to ten evacuations in one night. These could be bilious and yellow, dark brown and resembled an infusion of coffee in which floated small portions of stewed beef that had been over boiled. Cures tried are listed in considerable detail and the formulae for many of these are recorded. Recommendations, for example, to relieve headache and vertigo included immersing the legs in hot water mixed with two ounces (50 grams) of mustard flour for twenty minutes at bedtime. For diarrhoea, however, our learned friend was sceptical whether any 'ordinary, though potent, astringent medicine, would check it.'[29]

Having then looked at the outbreak in some detail, and identified the symptoms, we are now ready to answer the initial question: was this outbreak caused by the typhus microbe? I suggest, after consulting three doctors and from my own reading, that it was not.[30] This was, I believe, a typhoid epidemic caused by the polluted water that was drawn from the local wells and streams. The victims exhibited symptoms in a pattern that correlates with that disease. Symptoms that are recorded in lists of clinical features currently available to today's medical profession include: apathy, 'pea soup' or similar diarrhoea, abdominal distension, a cough, delirium and rambling talk, bradycardia (slow heart action) and pyrexia (fever).[31] Typhus also tended to be an endemic disease, whereas typhoid outbreaks were usually of an epidemic nature.

By 14 February 1844 the epidemic, begun the previous September, was over. It had resulted in fifty-one cases, eight of which proved to be fatal. There were, surprisingly, no cases amongst the, admittedly small, number of people over the age of fifty. We have already referred to the cruel lives of those living in nineteenth century towns where poor housing, overcrowding, inadequate sanitation and poverty was endemic. Those conditions were however, as we have seen, exhibited here in the Calder Valley and the typhoid outbreak had an equally devastating effect on the small community. To put what appears to be a small number of deaths in Slack in perspective it may be worth comparing the percentage of such with, say, Leeds in 1832. By extrapolating the 2.2 per cent death rate figures, a death toll of 1,672 would emerge!

Chapter Five

A Farmer, a Hired Man and a Milk Round

The 1880-81 Halifax Scarlet Fever Epidemic

Towards the end of 1880, and during the first two months of 1881, there was a serious and frightening outbreak of scarlet fever in Halifax. It affected a total of at least 510 people and there were 102 deaths from the disease. It reached its peak during the second week of January, when 188 people across all classes were infected.[1] This, however, was no ordinary outbreak and what makes it especially interesting is the debate that centred upon the source of the disease, and its spread through infected milk. It involved, as we shall see, a farmer, a hired man and a local milk round.

Scarlet fever, often also referred to as scarlatina, (the terms are interchangeable) was one of the chief epidemic diseases of the nineteenth and early twentieth centuries, with many lethal outbreaks in Halifax and across the country. It is an acute and chiefly childhood disease, caused by haemolytic streptococcal infection of the throat, skin or middle ear. It has a particularly short incubation period of usually two to three days within a range of one to eight. The symptoms vary but usually the patient experiences nausea, headache and shivers. A red rash often occurs and this is the symptom that gives the disease its name. It is usually spread, as in the case of a number of other diseases, by close contact and droplet infection but can also, according to F. B. Smith, be carried in clothes, dishes and even bedroom dust. Occasionally, and here we have a link with the Halifax outbreak, it can breed rapidly in milk or food handled by an infected person.[2] This, it was found, was the case in the Halifax outbreak.

The disease was viewed with dread, especially by parents with children under the age of ten. Although all ages could contract the disease and die from the infection, 95 per cent of cases were children up to the age of ten and the chances of them dying from the disease were high.[3] Arthur Whitelegge, who was the West Riding County MOH from 1889-1896,[4] gave a case mortality figure of ten per cent as a 'fair average'. It could be so deadly that it destroyed life in a few days, 'sometimes even in a few hours'.[5] It was, therefore, not difficult to imagine how parents in Halifax felt when they read in the *Halifax Guardian* on 8 January 1881 that 'a very serious outbreak of scarlet fever has occurred in the upper portion of the town'.[6]

They would know from hearing of other epidemics across the country, and from deaths within their own families and amongst friends, just how fearsome the

Cruel Lives

disease could be. The first great outbreak of the disease all over England was in 1840 followed by periodic national outbreaks throughout the century. In 1863, in England and Wales, over 34,000 had died from scarlet fever and in 1874, the figure was 26,000. In 1870, for example, it had been responsible for 6.5 per cent of all deaths in England and Wales.[7] In 1877 there had been one hundred deaths from the disease in Halifax [8] and in 1879 scarlet fever had killed 184 people in nearby Bradford.[9]

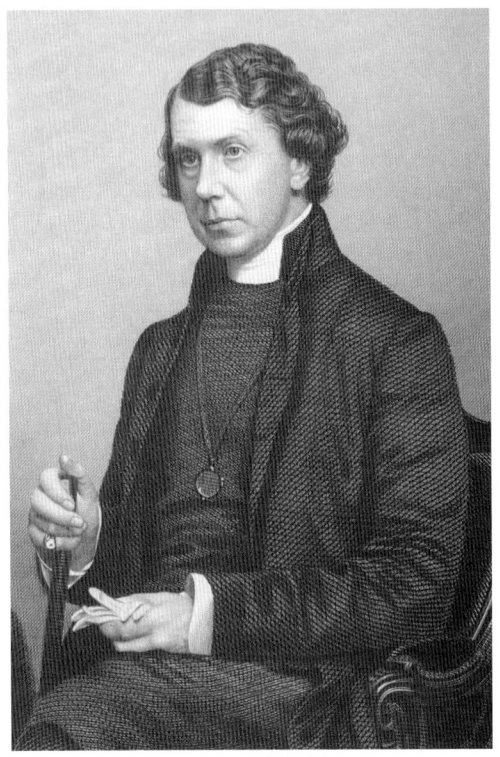

Figure 5:1 Archibald Tait: Archbishop of Canterbury 1868-1882
(The Bridgeman Art Gallery, London)
When Dean of Carlisle he lost five daughters to scarlet fever in the spring of 1856

The people of Halifax may also have read in August of the following year, 1880, just five months before the Halifax outbreak, the quite dreadful news relating to the station master of the Midland Railway in Bradford. In a period of eight days Robert Smith and his wife had lost all their four children to the disease. Horace and Ralph aged nine years and one year respectively had died on 3 August, Godfrey, four, on 8 August, and Rowland who was seven, two days later.[10] There had also been a similar case in Carlisle in 1856 when Archibald Tait, then the Dean of Carlisle but destined for the highest position in the Anglican Church, and his wife Catherine lost five of their daughters to scarlet fever in less than one month during March and early April. Charlotte was the first to die on 6 March, followed by Susan Elizabeth, Frances Alice, Catherine Anna, and finally Mary Susan on 8 April. One child, a son Craufurd, did survive. Three more daughters, Lucy, Edith and Agnes had, however, been born by April 1861. Tait became Bishop of London in November of 1856, a mere seven months after the loss of his daughters. In 1868 he was enthroned as Archbishop of Canterbury, a position he held until his death in December 1882.[11]

Doctors nationally were soon to learn from the *British Medical Journal (BMJ)* on 22 January that, following the sudden outbreak in Halifax, the disease was spreading in the town with 'alarming rapidity'.[12] The outbreak was, in fact, so sudden that the Halifax Medical Officer of Health, Dr. Daniel Ainley, was certain that it pointed *prima facie* to some common source. His foresight was eventually proved to be correct when within three days of the outbreak he was, he reported, able to discover the source and arrest it.[13] The outbreak was, he believed, to be the result of the distribution of milk from a farm outside the borough by a farmer who had scarlatina in his family. This 'beyond all question', he reported, was the cause of the outbreak but there were those, as we shall see, who took very strong exception to this assertion.[14] His conclusion was based on the simple premise that, as so many cases had quickly occurred in such a small cluster of houses, the outbreak pointed to 'one common cause'.[15]

Of the four short-listed likely candidates: the air, the drains, the water and the milk he selected milk as the villain. The *BMJ* was, however, more cautious when it reported on 22 January that 'various speculations are rife as to the causation of the outbreak' although it did add that the milk supply was, amongst other matters, was 'being impugned'.[16] On 12 February it reiterated the point that Dr. Ainley's conclusion is 'disputed by other inquirers into the circumstances'. It was important, all were agreed, that as 'fully a tenth' of all cases had proved to be fatal, the cause of this widely spread infection should be cleared up as soon as possible.[17]

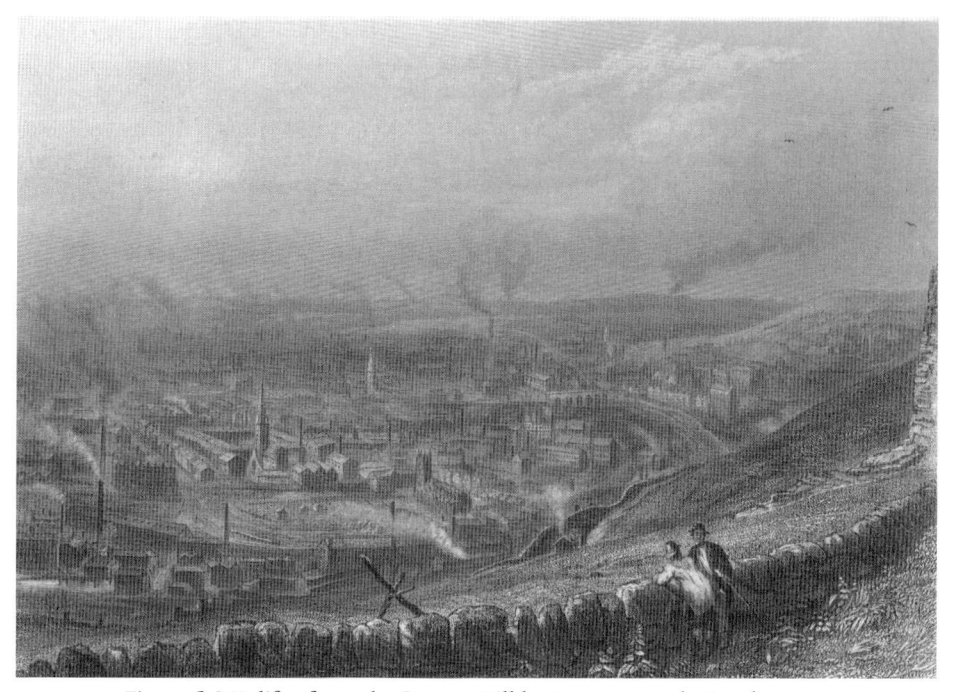

Figure 5:2 Halifax from the Beacon Hill by N Warren and J Stephenson.
(Calderdale MBC: Communities Directorate: Cultural Services)

This late nineteenth-century depiction of Halifax shows Halifax at its 'smoke enshrouded worst'.[18] Edward Wadsworth, the artist, (see chapter six) commented 'it's like hell isn't it', when looking down from Beacon Hill with Percy Wyndham Lewis in 1920.[19]

Charles Creighton, writing in 1884, makes it clear that ' there can be no question' milk and cream have been the vehicles of scarlatinal infection. Many outbreaks, he records, had been amongst the inmates of houses supplied with milk from a common source. In fact in 1881 at least fifteen outbreaks of the disease in Great Britain had been attributed to milk.[20] He also refers to a 'remarkable case' in which a large number of guests at an evening party, who had eaten strawberries and cream, were then attacked with scarlet fever at their respective homes.[21] This

Cruel Lives

information bears a strong resemblance to a gathering in Halifax that I refer to later. This view was also presented in the *BMJ* when it quoted the work of Sir Thomas Watson. He had indicated that scarlet fever was extremely subtle and tenacious; it can 'lurk about an apartment and cling to furniture and clothes for a very long time'. Its activity did, however, seem to depend on the medium that conveys it and milk, he suggested, 'increased the life and energy of its passenger'. He used an outbreak in Fallowfield, near Manchester in 1879 to support his views.[22]

Initial Suspicions

The initial outbreak in Halifax occurred in the upper part of Hopwood Lane where seventy cases were quickly identified. On Monday 3 January the medical officer had been informed that Robert Bell, a farmer in a 'small way' at Royles (Roils) Head with around six cows, who sold the milk in that locality, and also two gallons a day to the military canteen, was ill at home.[23] The farmer also purchased milk from three adjoining farms when he found that his own supply was not 'equal to the demands for it'.[24] When the sanitary inspector visited the farm later that day, he found that Bell's son, Thomas, who had been responsible for the distribution of some of the milk, was also ill with some form of sore throat. Suspicions were, no doubt, immediately aroused but as he had only been ill since the previous Saturday he could not have been responsible for the outbreak. Nor could the three other farmers who supplied milk for Bell's milk round, as their cows' milk was also found to be clear following a visit from the inspector.[25]

What could not be discounted, even at this at this early stage, was the role of a 'certain hired man' who had helped with the distribution of milk since October

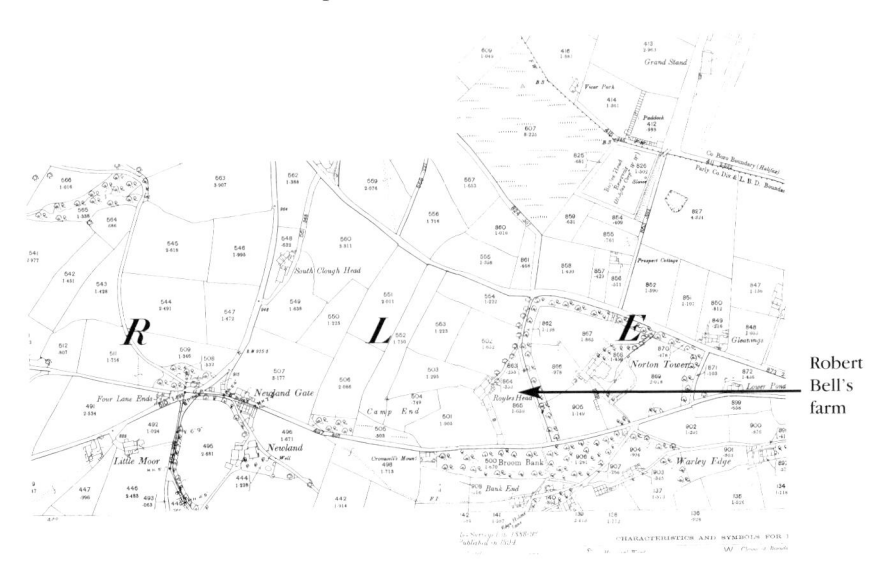

Figure 5:3 The location of the homes of Robert Bell and William Horsfield.
(Ordnance Survey 1894 surveyed 1888-1893, sheets CCXXX 7&8. Original scale1:2500)

The distance from Newland Gate, where Horsfield lived, to Bell's farm was approximately just over one-third of a mile (0.5km)

and, following the son's illness, carried out the task on his own. This had occurred in relation to both deliveries on Christmas Day and again during the first five days of January. The milk, it is important to remember, would have been ladled from a large container into jugs on the doorstep, with a hand-dipper. The man, described as an unpleasant person by the name of William Horsfield, lived 'very uncleanly' with his wife, Mary, and six children in a small cottage at Newlands in the village of Warley.

When the Medical Officer of Health and the inspector visited Horsfield's home, they found four children in one bed covered only by a single blanket and a bundle of rags, all suffering from scarlet fever. The house was 'very dirty' and the inspector found it to be so offensive that he cut short his visit there.[26] The eldest child, a daughter, was away working at a mill in Luddenden[27] but the other five children aged eight, six, three and one (the age of the other child is not recorded in the reports but the 1881 census shows another three year old in the family) were, or would be, attacked with the disease between 31 December and 14 January. Here, said Dr. Ainley, was the clue to the whole.[28] Owing to the man's 'household arrangements', he reported later, he could not have failed to attach 'contagious material to his person'.[29]

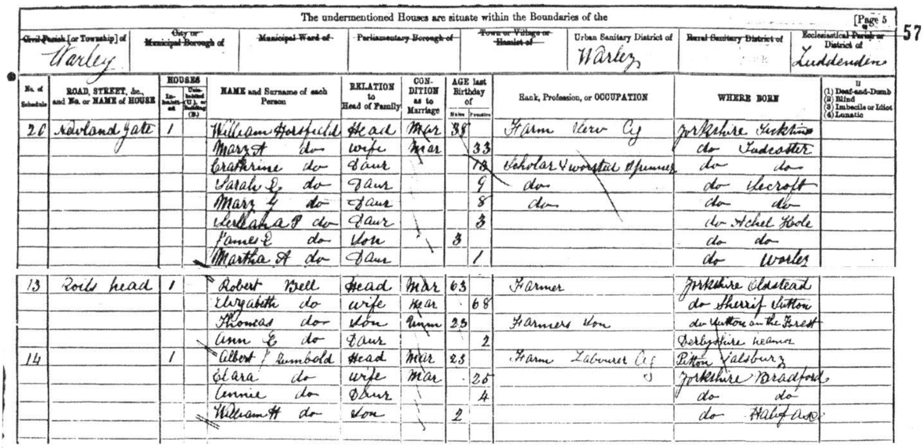
The undermentioned Houses are situate within the Boundaries of the [Page 5 57

Civil Parish [or Township] of Warley | City or Municipal Borough of | Municipal Ward of | Parliamentary Borough of | Town or Village or Hamlet of | Urban Sanitary District of Warley | Rural Sanitary District of | Ecclesiastical Parish or District of Luddenden

No. of Schedule	ROAD, STREET, &c., and No. or NAME of HOUSE	HOUSES Inhabited	HOUSES Uninhabited (U.), or Building (B.)	NAME and Surname of each Person	RELATION to Head of Family	CONDITION as to Marriage	AGE last Birthday of Males	AGE last Birthday of Females	Rank, Profession, or OCCUPATION	WHERE BORN	(1) Deaf-and-Dumb (2) Blind (3) Imbecile or Idiot (4) Lunatic
20	Newland Gate	1		William Horsfield	Head	Mar	38		Farm Serv Ag	Yorkshire Tockwith	
				Mary A do	wife	Mar		33		do Tadcaster	
				Cathrine do	daur			13	Scholar & worsted spinner	do do	
				Sarah E do	daur			9	do	do Tecroft	
				Mary J do	daur			8	do	do do	
				[illegible] do	daur			3		do Achel Hole	
				James E do	Son		3			do do	
				Martha A do	daur			1		do Warley	
13	Roils head	1		Robert Bell	Head	Mar	63		Farmer	Yorkshire Oldstead	
				Elizabeth do	wife	Mar		68		do Sherrif Sutton	
				Thomas do	Son	Unm	23		Farmers Son	do Sutton on the Forest	
				Ann E do	daur			2		Derbyshire [illegible]	
14		1		Albert J Rumbold	Head	Mar	23		Farm Labourer Ag	Pitton Salisbury	
				Clara do	wife	Mar		25		Yorkshire Bradford	
				Lennie do	daur			4		do do	
				William H do	Son		2			do Halifax	

Figure 5:4 1881 census showing the Bell and Horsfield families.

The man had gone each day from his home infected in 'person and clothing alike' with the 'most contagious and fatal disease', to milk the cows at Bell's farm and in doing so convey the germs to the milk that he would later distribute with a hand-dipper within the locality.[30] Horsfield's household arrangements were elaborated in the *BMJ* on 12 February. The man, it was suggested, would have had to attend to all his wife's household duties and do what nursing he could. We also get a fascinating account of the bedtime arrangements regarding Horsfield's clothes. As was the 'invariable rule in persons of his class', he would put all his clothes on the bed for extra warmth. Dr. Ainley believed, even at this early stage, that:

Beyond all doubt the cause of the outbreak is the distribution of milk by a certain hired man.[31]

Cruel Lives

The first forty cases were confined, with one exception, to the people in the neighbourhood of Craven Terrace and the top of Hopwood Lane who had their milk supplied from this source.[32] During the following week the disease spread to other areas and the *Halifax Guardian* reported on 15 January that:

The outbreak of scarlet fever, mentioned last week as having occurred in the upper portion of the town has, since Saturday, spread with alarming rapidity, entering the houses of rich and poor alike, visiting neighbourhoods supposed to be the most salubrious in Halifax, laying the children prostrate with fever, and producing in adults a painful disease of the throat.[33]

The *Halifax Courier*, a weekly paper in those days, as it is again in 2012, supported this view and informed readers that the number of cases reported by the sanitary authority at the Town Hall by Thursday, 13 January had risen to a total of 179. Many cases had, it was regretted, not been reported. Those recorded were identified as 121 cases of scarlet fever and fifty-eight of scarlatina sore throat. Here we find an interesting separation of the two terms, scarlet fever and scarlatina. The suffering of some families had, reported the paper, been very great. At one house, in Norfolk Place, five members of the family were infected with scarlatina and three with a sore throat. It was also reported that a respected minister has also one case of scarlet fever and four of sore throat in his family.[34]

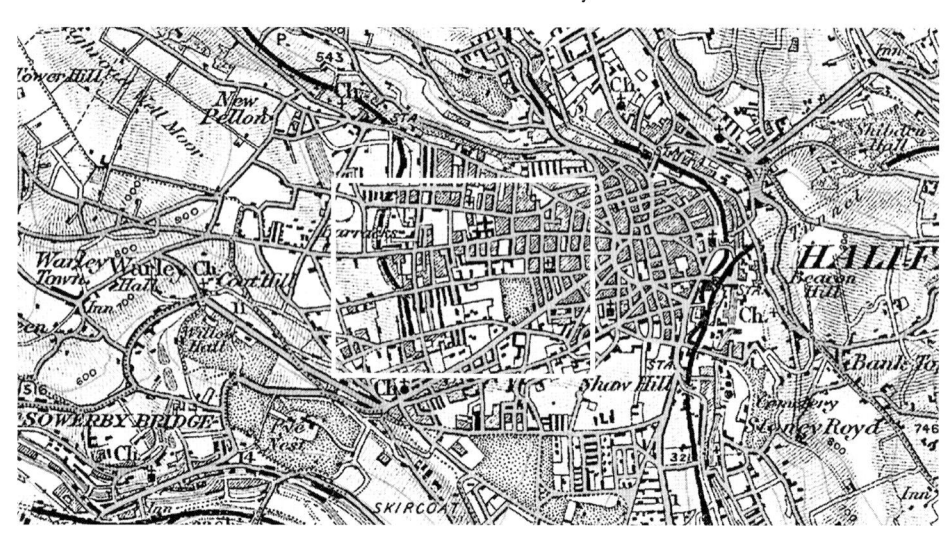

Figure 5:5 The area to the west of the town, where the outbreak was centred.
(Cassini Historical Map 104. Revised New Series. 1903-1904.)

Details relating to deaths from the disease first appeared in both the local papers on 15 January. The *Halifax Guardian* notes that in twelve of the cases fateful results have occurred, whereas the *Halifax Courier* has the figure at thirteen. The latest deaths were to the west of the town centre at Aspinall Street and Vickerman Street, adjacent streets off Hopwood Lane, and Gerrard Street off Gibbet Street (see figure 5:5). The number of deaths to date was reported to be rather low indicating, readers were informed, that the disease was of a mild nature. Despite this apparent optimism, by the following week on 22 January the *Halifax Courier* was reporting that the number of cases had risen by seventy and that the death toll had increased by thirteen bringing the total to twenty-six. However, there had been 'a great decline' in the number of new cases. It was also encouraging to note, the paper said, that the area under infection, chiefly South Ward, had scarcely extended at all. Alongside this information it was noted that scarlet fever had reached Wood Hall, Copley Wood and Underbank, Sowerby Bridge. The disease was, it was suggested, being checked by the precautions being taken by the sanitary authorities and the public. They were aided by the high winds and sharp frosts of the week.[35]

On 29 January the public learned that, although the weekly death toll was decreasing, there was still the need for great caution, especially as the weather was no longer of a 'favourable character'. The thick fogs were such as to try the constitutions of the 'most strong'.[36] The number of cases had risen to 335 of which 233 were scarlet fever and the rest sore throat, referred to as scarlatina in previous reports. The death toll had also risen to thirty-five with nine new cases.[37] Little information is given throughout the newspaper reports in relation to the victims; their names, their ages and their addresses. The *Halifax Guardian* of 22 January did, however, provide a small amount of information relating to the victims. There had been five instances since the epidemic began, where two deaths had appeared in one house: in Gibbet Street, Bull Green, Craven Terrace, Coton (sic) Street and Vickerman Street.[38] No names or actual addresses are provided.

However, my research into St Paul's Church, King Cross, burial records has unearthed information relating to the family of Edward Gledhill, a thirty-year-old bank clerk, and his family. They lived at 126 Queens Road, also listed as Ashfield Terrace in the 1881 Kelly's Directory.[39] The church register shows that between 13 - 31 January 1881 there were eleven burials, all were of children aged five years and under. The overwhelming majority of these deaths were, I suggest, as a direct result of the scarlet fever epidemic. Two of them were the children of Edward and Mary Louise Gledhill. Arthur was buried on 15 January aged seven months and Thomas, aged five, followed nine days later.[40] Their second child, Albert, survived the epidemic. Sadness, however, continued to follow Edward as his wife died in 1888, aged thirty-seven, and he passed away in 1899 aged forty-eight.[41]

Differing Opinions

The preventative measures taken by the local authority quickly came under scrutiny once the epidemic had started to subside. Scott believed that 'beyond prohibition of the infected carrier from distributing the milk', little in the way of preventative measures was undertaken.[42] The epidemic was, in his view, an example of how a contagious disease could be spread by a mismanaged milk business. This may, on reflection, appear somewhat harsh as the newspaper reports indicate that some effort was made to prevent the spread of the disease. On 15 January the sanitary inspector Mr. Travis and his sub-inspector, Mr. Hoyle, were reported to be working from morning until late at night to ascertain the state of the drains, giving advice, and taking prompt sanitary measures. Chloride of lime was distributed 'gratuitously' from the Town Hall and the drains flushed in Bentley

Cruel Lives

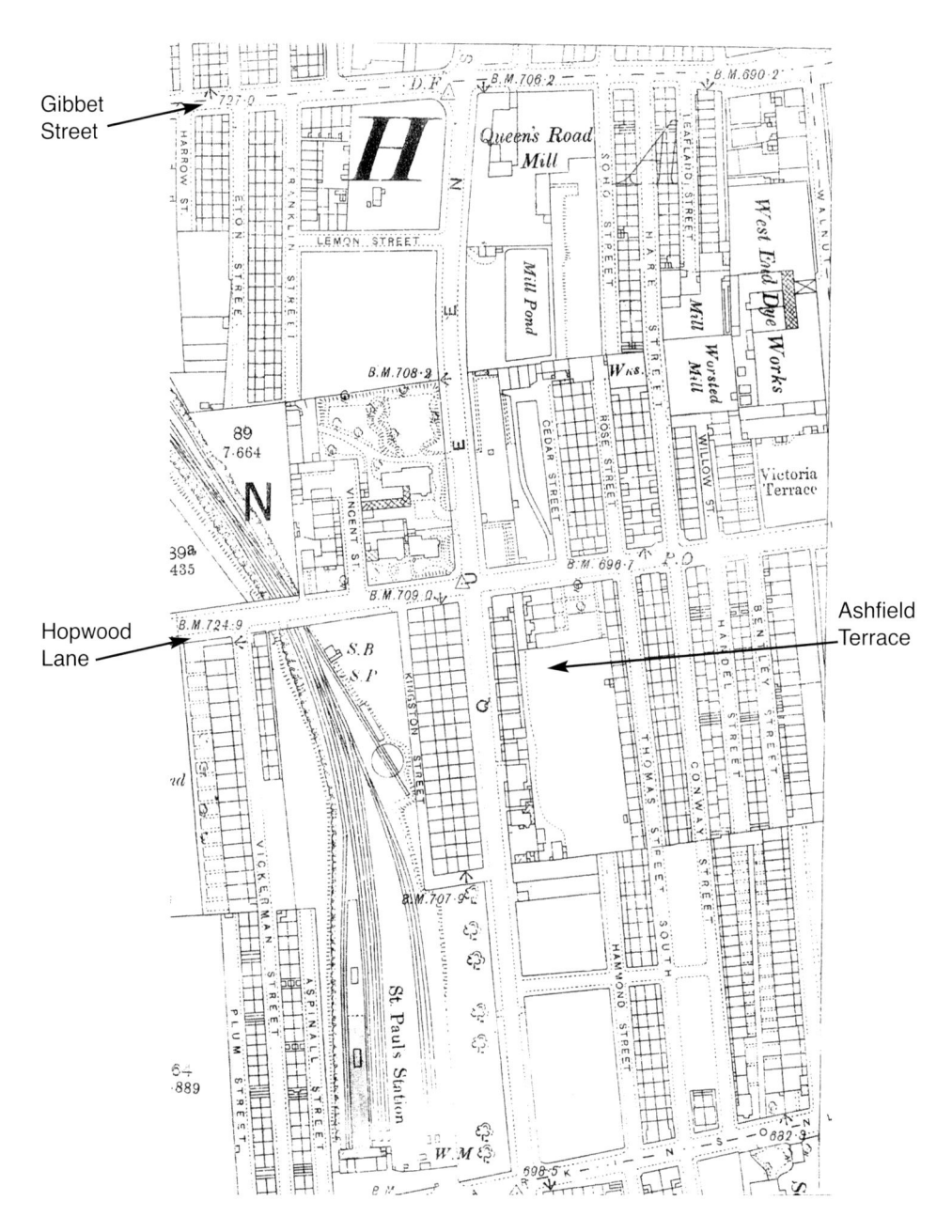

Figure 5:6 The area around the junction of Hopwood Lane and Queen Street, where a number of deaths occurred.
(Ordnance Survey Map published 1894, surveyed 1888-92. Original scale 1:2500.)

St Paul's Station, across the road from Ashfield Terrace, was the terminus of the Great Northern Halifax High level Railway. The branch line left the Queensbury line from Halifax North Bridge Station at Holmfield.

Street and Hopwood Lane. The Goux closets* had been emptied every other day and handbills giving advice regarding matters of cleanliness and isolation had been distributed. Farmers and milk dealers had been visited to check whether any germs of disease had been conveyed in the water. W. H. Wood, the Borough Analyst, was able to report on 12 January that water from the Victoria reservoir was 'free from contamination of organic matter' and again two days later that the water was free from any sewage contamination.[43] The *Halifax Courier* was confident that everything possible was being done when it reported that 'the authorities are adopting every possible means of stamping out the disease'.[44]

There were many, however, who had other views on how the disease was spread. The water supply was questioned and, as we shall see, was the subject of a lengthy report by the MOH. The water supply was checked throughout the epidemic and all the reports were that water from the local reservoirs at Victoria and Roils Head was free from contamination with sewage or any dangerous organic matter. Sewage was blamed by others. A correspondent wrote to the *Halifax Courier* to say that 'an eminent doctor, talking to a friend this week', had said that it was not the milkman at all who was to blame 'but sewage gas and nothing else'.[45]

Day schools and Sunday Schools, were closed once the outbreak had taken a grip on the community. The *Halifax Guardian* reported on 22 January that the bellman had been round on Saturday, 15 January making announcements in relation to which Sunday Schools were closed. The long list in the paper gives some indication of the strength of the Sunday School movement at that time. The day schools closed, the paper reported, included Queens Road, St Augustine's and Pellon Lane.[46] Head teachers also recorded the progress of the epidemic and the school closures in their log books. On 14 January the head of Halifax Parish Church National School notes that the fever is 'very rife' in parts of the town and, a week later, that 'much fear is excited' by the rapid spread of the disease. Although this school appears to have avoided initial closure, when a case of scarlet fever was reported in one pupil's house on 31 January, the school closed.[47]

At Queen's Road Board School we read that the school closed on Friday 11 January for two weeks, and at the adjacent Girls' School closure occurred on the following Monday.[48] At Pellon Lane Infants' School, where closure was announced from 17 January until 1 February, owing to the 'epidemic of scarlet fever and scarlatina' the headteacher also recorded that Walter and Percy Gledhill had been sent home at 11am because of their brother having typhoid fever.[49] Pupils could clearly be sent home immediately a problem arose and there were not the procedures in place that would apply today. An example of a sudden and emergency closure is noted in the Pellon Lane School Boys' Department on 17 January, when the head teacher recorded that:

We had got prayers over and the registers partly called, when the clerk to the School Board came and ordered us to close the school for a fortnight on account

---

* The Goux closet was the invention of Frenchman Pierre Nicholas Goux. The system consisted of a pail lined with absorbent material. When collected, perhaps on a weekly basis, the pails were immediately replaced with a clean and empty one.[53]

of scarlet fever in the town. The lads were accordingly sent home.[50]

> Jany 19th & 21st
>
> We had got prayers over and the registers partly called when the clerk to the School Board came and ordered us to close school for a fortnight on account of Scarlet Fever in the town. The lads were accordingly sent home.
>
> 201

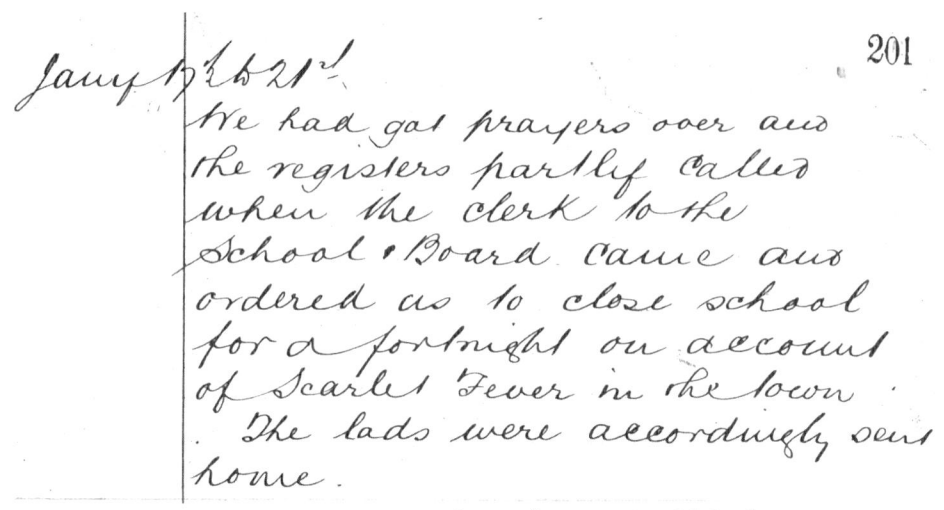

Figure 5:7 Log book entry from Pellon Lane Boys' School.
(West Yorkshire Archive Service, Calderdale. Ref:OR/ED 255a(i))

Closure of schools for lengthy periods during epidemics was, of course, a regular occurrence at this time as they were a rich breeding ground for infectious outbreaks. A trawl through almost any school log book shows closures for local outbreaks of measles and chicken pox and occasionally for more serious diseases such as smallpox and diphtheria.[51] Even when epidemics had subsided, parents were often reluctant to send their children back to school. When Queen's Road Board School reopened on 1 February, we read that many parents still refused to send their children to school on account of the fever, a note repeated a week later. At the Girls' School many children were still absent as late as the 15 February.[52]

As well as the school closures, Sunday school, and day schoolmasters and superintendents were also encouraged to follow the example set at an examination on 13 January. Those present were asked to show, by raising their hands, if scarlet fever was present in their homes. Two children did so and were sent home. Night schools at the Mechanics' Institute had also closed. Public gatherings in the Borough had ceased and the Yeomanry Cavalry ball had been postponed.[54] Some public libraries closed and where they remained open notices were displayed telling people not to return books from infected homes. In addition printed bills were distributed to every house giving details of the symptoms and 'both restorative and preventative information' relating to every stage of the disease.[55]

One of the most fertile ways of spreading the infection was children's parties, reported the *Courier*, and the readers, it was suggested, would no doubt hope that these were also cancelled or postponed. A great deal with regard to prevention clearly depended on the people themselves. They were encouraged to boil milk and to act in a responsible manner with regard to reporting outbreaks. Although visiting from house to house was actively discouraged in the infected district, the doctors who continued with their work and passed from house to house, 'without taking any precautions whatsoever', were praised by the *Halifax Courier*.[56] There were, inevitably, some cases where the public had displayed gross carelessness in homes where the fever prevailed.[57]

On 1 February the *Halifax Courier* reported that there had been very few new cases during the week but this news did not dampen the opinions of the people. There continued to be discussions, and mixed views, relating to the role that the water supply may have played in the spread of the disease. Some of these views clearly still annoyed Dr. Ainley almost twelve months after the outbreak, as we shall hear. In a report to the Sanitary Committee he again reiterated his belief that 'beyond all question the outbreak was caused by the farmer's helper at Warley, who, whilst the fever was in his family continued to milk the cows and deliver the milk in the town'. He also described the means taken to arrest the outbreak. These included an early instruction to the farmer's man to refrain from attending to his normal duties, and a house-to-house canvass to ascertain who had been affected. Additionally he included a number of suggestions regarding any future outbreaks. One was that both money and sorrow would have been saved if the wages of the man who is 'supposed to have spread the disease' had been paid for him to stay at home.[58]

Table 5:1 Total number of cases reported: 1 November 1880-26 February 1881.

510 in 281 families (106 classed as 'well-to-do' families)
347 cases occurred in the South Ward
102 in the West Ward
18 in Skircoat Ward
16 in Central Ward
15 in Market Ward
12 unknown

A second point concerned the powers relating to the isolation of victims. Not until these were in line with the powers linked to the isolation of animals suffering from contagious diseases, would scarlet fever be stamped out. Isolation was the key to containment as there was little else in the way of treatment. An isolation hospital had been established at Stoney Royd in 1872 ostensibly for the isolation of smallpox and typhoid victims. It was, however, also used for the isolation of, for example, diphtheria and scarlet fever patients. In 1881 thirty-four cases of scarlet fever were admitted to Stoney Royd but little information relating to them or the hospital was reported in the local papers.[59] Some doctors had, in the past, suggested that there was 'seldom any occasion for medicine in this disease'. Even beyond the date of the Halifax outbreak doctors were still only recommending, 'general evacuants' to ease the ulceration of the throat, and copious bloodletting to lessen the 'unquestionable oppression of internal organs'.[60]

His final suggestion referred to the prompt application of a clause in the 1878 Contagious Diseases (Animals) Act that covered Dairies, Cowsheds and Milk Shops Order.[61] This was quickly acted upon when Henry Robinson, the meat inspector, was given greater powers and was to inspect all registered farms.[62] By the middle

Cruel Lives

of the nineteenth century there had been growing concern about the state of sanitation on dairy farms. The milk was untreated and often outbreaks of disease were blamed on milk-houses.[63] In fact, indicated Dr. Ainley, no article of general consumption was so dangerous to the health of people as milk.[64] He received support for his views relating to the water supply from Dr. Thomas Britton, in whose health district the man (Horsfield) who milked the cows lived, in a piece published in the *Halifax Guardian* on 29 January. Thomas Britton, who also acted as MOH for Brighouse, was himself to fall victim of an epidemic, this time influenza, and died the following year on 29 December.[65] He wrote to the mayor as follows:

I have been informed that the idea has become current in the town to the effect that I ascribe the fever now prevailing to the drinking of water from the fly reservoir. The water in question cannot possibly have caused the fever.

He then went on to explain that it was desirable that all drinking water should be free from both animal and vegetable contamination especially when an epidemic was present. For that reason only did he recommend boiling the water prior to it being used for drinking purposes and not because he had any fear that that it would cause scarlatina. The paper somewhat sarcastically suggested that readers were 'at liberty to make what use they like of the letter'.[66]

Thomas Britton may have been clarifying his position or had he changed his mind? He must, therefore, have been annoyed when he read his copy of the *BMJ* on 19

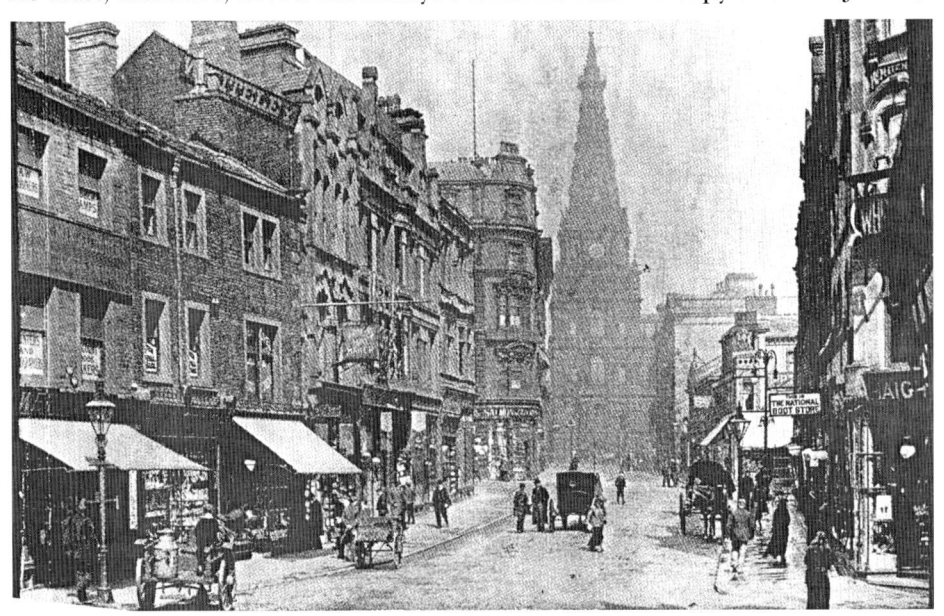

Figure 5:8 Halifax c1890
(Calderdale MBC, Communities Directorate: Cultural Services)

The town centre from Southgate. The fine Town Hall, designed by Sir Charles Barry and opened in 1863, looks down on this late nineteenth-century scene from the head of Princess Street.[67] Only six deaths from scarlet fever occurred in the Central Ward.

February. The journal, admittedly not as up to date with its news as a local paper, was still indicating that 'Dr. Britton denies that the man could have caused the mischief' and had suggested that he contracted the disease in Halifax. His arguments, the journal believed, 'were not very cogent'![68]

The *Halifax Guardian* did, however, have good news for the people of Halifax when it reported on 12 February that 'the epidemic of scarlatina which has prevailed amongst us some weeks appears to be gradually dying out [and] we are glad to note that an inspector is to be "sent down" at an early date'.[69]

The Official Inquiry

This evidence in Dr. Ainley's report had, then, resulted in the Local Government Board asking a Dr. Ballard to carry out an official enquiry. This news clearly pleased, amongst others, the editor of the *BMJ* and the journal reported on 19 February that:

We are glad to be in a position to state that the Local Government Board have acceded to the request made to them by a number of medical practitioners and other residents of Halifax, for an enquiry by one of the Board's medical staff.[70]

Dr. Ballard, who led the inquiry, had completed it by April and was able later that month to attend a special meeting of the Halifax Town Council to make a statement relating to his enquiries. These corroborated the MOH's views to a certain extent but he did not consider that the distribution of milk was the cause of the first introduction of the disease into the town. Scarlet fever, he indicated, had been constantly appearing – sometimes in one district, sometimes in another. Readers will also recall that the eldest child of Horsfield, a daughter, was working at a mill in Luddenden when the inspector first called at his home. Scott suggests that she could well have conveyed the disease to other members of her family as there were cases of scarlet fever in Luddenden during November 1880.[71]

The statistical evidence presented by Ballard was extremely detailed, although the accuracy of the information passed on to him was questioned by some people. Indeed, in a letter to the *Halifax Guardian* on 29 January a local general practitioner, Dr. Dolan of Horton House, suggested that the returns were not accurate.[72] It is difficult not to agree with this view as the milkman kept no books and his trade was very much on a 'ready money' basis as, perhaps, we would expect. To be fair, however, when an inquiry was made from house to house, few errors were detected in the list that had been compiled from memory by Robert Bell and his son Thomas.

The milk dealer had supplied 135 families, and 125 were traced and interviewed. By 14 February, fifty-three families had provided one or more patients who had had some form of the disease. The seventy-two who escaped 'invasion' were broken down as follows. Twenty-nine households contained adults only who were less susceptible to the disease and were, perhaps, not drinking milk to the same degree as children. Fifteen others had children who had all previously been infected; in a further seven the majority of children in the household had previously had the disease; and in seven more no accurate information could be obtained. In fourteen 'clear' homes only, could he find that no one had previously had the disease. In these households two families boiled the milk and in a further family one had stopped taking milk deliveries owing to the dirty state of the man. He also raised the question of natural immunity when indicating that in another two households three generations had not had the disease.[73] Is there, asks Scott, natural immunity to scarlet fever?[74]

Table 5:2 Survey of distribution of milk from Robert Bell's farm
135 households supplied; 125 traced and of these:
- 53 provided more than one patient.
- 72 escaped invasion and these can be broken down further as follows:
  29 households occupied by adults only,
  15 had children living in them who had already had scarlet fever,
  7 where no accurate information was obtained,
  14 where no-one had suffered from SF (two boiled their milk, one had stopped deliveries recently owing to the filthy state of 'the man')

At a distance of over a hundred years this appears to be pretty conclusive but clearly the doctor wanted even harder evidence and his epidemiological research took him a stage further. (see table 5:3). He took a sample of thirteen streets in which the milk supply of each house was ascertained. Eighty-two families were supplied by Robert Bell, and a further 188 by a variety of local milkmen. Of the eight-two who were Bell's customers, forty-five were infected with scarlet fever whereas only fourteen of the other 188 households were attacked.

Table 5:3 Further research was conducted amongst a sample of 13 streets and in these:
82 families received milk from Bell and here there were 45 cases of SF (54.9% attack rate)
188 received milk from other suppliers. 14 cases of SF occurred here (7.4% attack rate)

In four of the streets investigated there was only one household in each receiving milk from Bell. There were SF sufferers in all four houses: one following the Christmas period, three in the first week in January.

Of the forty-five cases in the first group, all had occurred before 9 January, whereas only three of the fourteen in the second group had been infected before that date. The importance of that particular date in relation to the son's illness and the sanitary authority stopping the hired man from delivering milk on 5 January was emphasised. Before giving guidance re future procedures Dr. Ballard also reported the 'curious case' of an outbreak amongst twenty-six of the thirty-five people who had attended a party in January. It transpired that the cream served had been obtained from a farm adjacent to Bell's at Warley.[75]

In his report he accepted that accumulations of infected filth are sometimes agents for the extension of the disease. He went on to make general points with regard to sewers, privies and water closets and noted that 'water closets are not habitually ventilated as they should be'. The inns and lodging-houses had been badly looked after during the outbreak. Medical men who refused information to the doctor were at fault and they should have sent a record of their cases to the sanitary authorities. The public were also at fault, but their fault was one of ignorance. He could, however, find no indications that scarlatina in Halifax was attributable to faulty sewers and drains. He closed his report with two further recommendations regarding isolation of cases and more systematic disinfection of properties affected. He believed that an order should be served on households, requiring cleansing of the premises and all things within that were capable of conveying infection.[76] There were, then, points for development but Dr. Ainley must surely have been reassured by what he heard.

What then are our final thoughts after over a hundred years? The evidence gathered in 1881 clearly points to the milk being delivered by Horsfield as the cause of the outbreak, but was he solely responsible? In 1934 Harold Scott argued that, although the hired man was a very active agent in spreading infection, it could be contracted independently. It did not follow, therefore, that he was the only source, or that he was responsible for the infection in all those who were supplied by him. However, it was shown that he had stopped delivering milk on 6 January and no further instances arose among the households receiving this milk more than three days after his deliveries ceased, a clear indication, it would appear, of his involvement in the outbreak. Some on the list could have acquired the infection through other means, such as direct contact and droplet infection, and some cases had been notified prior to the children of the distributor being infected. There were, suggests Scott, cases that clearly could not 'be ascribed, at any rate directly, to this man'.[77]

Many will argue, even today, that it is difficult from this distance to 'sentence' Horsfield. Was it the cows that were infected, possibly by Bell's son, and Horsfield was guilty only of delivering milk that was already infected? The multiplication of organisms is actually inhibited by the properties of raw milk, so contamination of milk by the carrier is considered unlikely to cause an outbreak.[78] Finally, did Horsfield himself infect the cows with his contaminated hands, when he began milking, and pass on the bacteria (possibly *Streptococcus pyogenes*) causing a lethal form of mastitis?

In other cases of milk-borne septic sore throat and scarlet fever, such as in New York and Vermont in 1893;[79] and in Doncaster in 1937, where there was an outbreak of milk borne scarlet fever and tonsillitis, there was more inconclusive evidence.[80] The outbreak in Doncaster that had 'several points of interest' was, it was agreed, due to infection of the milk with *Steptococcus pyogenes* and the primary infection appeared to be have been through the cow becoming infected. However, from the evidence 'obtainable locally' it was reported that the possibility of direct contamination of the milk by a milker could not be entirely disregarded. Two deaths were definitely associated with the outbreak: a two-year old child who died of scarlet fever, and a male aged thirty-three who later developed adenitis (severe inflammation of lymph nodes) after a severe attack of tonsillitis.[81] The outbreak in America was judged to be the result of the milk being infected before it left the cow rather than contamination of milk in the time between it leaving the cow and reaching the consumer.[82] Following an outbreak in Brighton in 1906, Sir Arthur Newsholme suspected that the milk had been infected on the farm rather than in transit as, unlike the situation here, customers of different suppliers were affected.[83]

At the end of the year, eight months after the epidemic had subsided, the MOH's report was presented to the Borough of Halifax. Dr. Ainley covered again, for the benefit of all present, the history of the Halifax epidemic before reminding the council, that he had indicated in an earlier paper that *prima facie* the outbreak had pointed to a common source. Others, however, had questioned his judgement and blamed some occult or strange atmospheric phenomenon. One critic, he reminded everyone, who was 'especially severe', suggested that the outbreak was linked to badly constructed sewers. Dr. Ainley was clearly still annoyed by such criticisms, and we read that he considered that such comments were all 'bare assertion, without one tittle of evidence'.[84]

The satisfaction Dr. Daniel Ainley, M.R.C.S., L.R.C.P Medical Officer of Health must have gained as he added his name to the report, and then presented it, can only be imagined!

Appendix

Key dates from 1 November, 1880

By 30 November 1880: One confirmed death from Scarlet fever (SF) on 1 November.
Prior to 25 December, and from 26-31: Thomas Bell delivers milk each morning and with William Horsfield each evening.
25 December: Horsfield alone responsible for both deliveries.
1-31 December: Six confirmed deaths from SF.
31 December: First diagnosis of SF at Horsfield's home.
1 January 1881: Thomas Bell suffering from a sore throat and stopped work.
1-5 January: Horsfield brought in to milk cows and also delivers milk alone.
1 or 2 January: A child of Horsfield's is confirmed as suffering from SF.
4-5 January: Two further cases of SF amongst Horsfield's children.
6 January: Horsfield prohibited from milking and delivering milk.
8 January: No further cases, with one exception, occurred amongst those households receiving milk from Bell's farm.
14 January: A fifth child at Horsfield's has SF.
1-31 January: 52 deaths from SF in Halifax
1-26 February: 28 deaths from SF in Halifax.

Deaths from Zymotic (Infectious) Diseases in the Borough of Halifax for the year ending 31 December 1881.

Ward	Population	Small pox	Measles	Scarlet fever	Diphtheria	Whooping cough	Fever	Diarrhoea
Ovenden	5387			3	1		2	
Northowram	7405			3		1		
North	5474			1			3	
Central	8569	1		6		4	6	1
West	14,227	1	2	28	1	1	2	1
South	10,691		1	53		1	1	2
Market	3816			1		2		
East	5330		1	3	1	1	2	1
Southowram	5777	4	2	2			4	1
Skircoat	6955			2	1	7	1	
	73,633	6	6	102*	4	17	21	6

* There were 21 deaths from scarlet fever in Halifax in 1882[85]

The infectious diseases accounted for 10.2% of all deaths. Pulmonary disease (bronchitis, consumption and pneumonia) was responsible for 31.0% of deaths (497 in total). The overall Borough death rate per thousand of the population was 21.4, with the highest figures of 28.1 in South Ward, 26.9 in West, and the lowest, 15.3, in Skircoat.[86]

Chapter Six
A Memorable Visitation
The 1891 Spen Valley Influenza Epidemic

During the spring of 1891 the Spen Valley district of Yorkshire was visited 'memorably' by an attack of Russian Influenza;[1] an influenza strain that was, during that period, to kill fifty-eight thousand Britons. The Spen Valley influenza epidemic only lasted for four weeks during the spring of 1891, but during that short period the disease held a powerful grip on the towns and villages of that part of Yorkshire. The disease also had a profound effect in the towns to the east of the area. These included Batley, Birstall and Dewsbury. This, then, is an account of how a closely knit group of small towns was affected by the deadly virus and its pneumonic complications.

Influenza, usually referred to simply as flu, is a highly infectious viral disease that affects the respiratory tract. It is usually a winter disease, although this was not the case in May 1891, as it requires relatively low temperatures for its propagation.[2] The virus was greatly encouraged, as we have seen with other diseases, by poor diet which lowered people's resistance, general social conditions and the damp houses in which so many lived. Unlike other viruses the influenza virus has a nasty habit of fighting back. It is able to dodge the immune system by changing its H and N (*haemagglutinin and neurominidase*) genes, and to re-infect.[3]

Mark Honigsbaum believes that the Russian flu pandemic that raged during the years 1889-1892, the one that is central to our story, awakened interest in the disease.[4] Before then, health officials had accepted influenza with resignation. The disease had circulated in the past and it is thought possible that the first outbreak in Europe occurred in 1173.[5] Nothing on the scale of the outbreak witnessed during the years immediately following 1889 had, however, been experienced before.

The first identifiable epidemic of any consequence in England appears to have been in 1510, although outbreaks of English sweat or sweating sickness may, in fact, have been influenza.[6] Severe outbreaks followed on seven occasions from 1658*, but before the 1889 epidemic doctors had often regarded the condition as relatively harmless.[7] Now they had little choice but to take it seriously, especially as doctors were beginning to notice the connection between the wave of so called

---
* In 1775, 1782, 1803, 1823, 1833, 1837 and 1847-8

Russian influenza, that began in St. Petersburg in December 1889, and a 'low and insidious form of pneumonia'.[8] Russia had already seen considerable outbreaks in the late 1880s and in St. Petersburg especially, every winter from 1885 through to 1888.[9]

Influenza had always baffled doctors and for much of the nineteenth century, suggests Smith, they could not decide whether it was a specific disease.[10] In the case of the lobar pneumonias that they were now seeing they also were not sure whether the cause was the microbe itself or secondary bacterias. The other alarming feature of the 1889-1892 outbreak was the way that it attacked those in the thirty to fifty years age group. During an attack of the usual seasonal flu the victims were usually found amongst the elderly and very young.[11] The virus was lethal and struck quickly. People were reported as going to work feeling well and being in a bad way by eleven o'clock. The symptoms included severe prostration, weakness, muscular pain, shivering and headache.

The epidemic came in three distinct waves but it was the second wave in the spring of 1891 that caused the most anxiety and resulted in most deaths. This pattern of a mild primary wave, followed by a severe one, was repeated during the even more severe world-wide 1918 'Spanish flu' epidemic when 228,000 Britons expired. It enveloped the world, writes Honigsbaum, like a great tidal wave. People had no idea where it came from or how to combat it.[12] The death toll included those who had survived the war but had not lived long enough, it was thought, to develop immunities acquired during previous epidemics. The huge crowds that attended the armistice celebrations increased the chances of the disease spreading.[13] Half of the victims were this time in the twenty to forty years age group and, again, the usual U shaped graph of fatalities now took a different shape – this time that of a W.[14]

The 1891 outbreak caused concern right across the country as it swept south along the Pennines to Sheffield and on to London. One of the first fatal victims was Archbishop Magee of York who was in the capital at the time. As Lords, Members of Parliament and the Prince of Wales were taken ill, fumigation squads were brought in to spray the Houses of Parliament. Of all the places infected, the people of Sheffield do appear to have suffered the most with the death rate during the first week of May reaching seventy per thousand, the highest rate in the town's history.[15] In England and Wales the death toll in relation to recorded influenza deaths was 'only' 4,523 but the virus was associated with many respiratory complications and was directly responsible for over twenty-seven thousand deaths.

Influenza is reported in The Spen Valley

The Spen Valley is an area in what used to be the West Riding of Yorkshire, now West Yorkshire. It is surrounded to the north by Bradford; to the east by Leeds and, as already indicated Dewsbury, to the south by Huddersfield, and to the west by Halifax. It comprises a number of towns and communities, namely Cleckheaton, Liversedge, Gomersal and Heckmondwike. In 1891 each of these places was, along with Birkenshaw, an individual local board with its own Medical Officer of Health.

In 1894, following the Local Government Act, they became urban district councils.[16] In 1915 Cleckheaton, Gomersal and Liversedge amalgamated to create Spenborough Urban District Council.

Figure 6:1 The location of the Spen Valley towns in relation to the major conurbations in West Yorkshire.

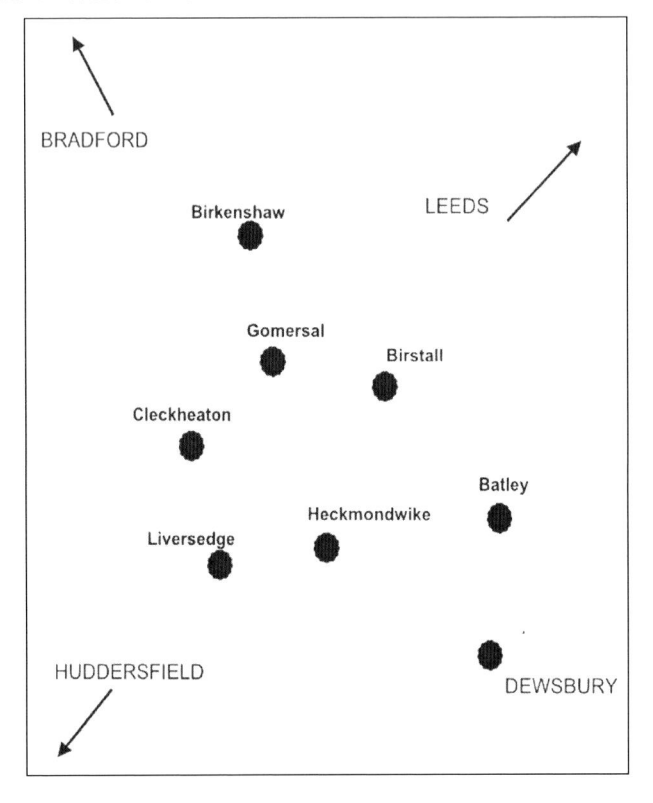

The first news of the outbreak in the north of England, where there had already been 375 deaths in Sheffield, reached the Spen Valley via the *Cleckheaton and Spen Valley Guardian* when, on 1 May, readers were informed that:

From all parts of the country reports come of the prevalence of influenza[17]

The disease had apparently, reported the *BMJ*, begun in Hull where cases had been recognised in February and became epidemic in March. From Hull, where numerous deaths had occurred from bronchitis and pneumonia,[18] the epidemic spread to the towns and villages in the neighbourhood. Driffield and Malton were attacked along with villages on both sides of the Humber.[19] In York three hundred men who worked at the North Eastern Railway's carriage sheds were absent with influenza. The papers were also quick to point out that the infectious disease was 'not a matter to be treated with levity' and that it closed schools and hindered industry.[20]

In the Spen Valley many people were already absent from work and doctors were busy 'in all directions'. There had been an increase in the number of death notices in the local paper on 1 May from thirty-four the previous week to fifty-seven;[21] a significant enough increase to cause, I am sure, some consternation amongst the medical profession.

There was, though, much optimism in the *Dewsbury Reporter* that circulated in the areas surrounding Dewsbury but also covered Heckmondwike. The disease was, it informed its readers, on 2 May, generally of a milder type than had previously been experienced. We learn, however, that the doctors were labouring with great assiduity and no lack of skill. No fatal results had been recorded in that area but a number of schools had closed. The situation to the west was clearly becoming more serious. It was 'raging' in Batley and 'prevalent' in Staincliffe. In Heckmondwike there was 'no abatement' in the epidemic and there and in Cleckheaton, where the doctors 'never were so busy as at present', two medical men had fallen victim to the complaint. The doctors were, apparently, 'run off their legs' and three deaths were, to date, attributed to influenza.[22] In Batley Dr. Swann reported that in all his experience he had never seen anything like it before. He and his assistant Dr. Stewart had 300 cases to attend.[23]

A week later the situation was deeply worrying. 'Extraordinary Mortality in Heckmondwike' was the headline that greeted readers of the *Cleckheaton and Spen Valley Guardian*. The paper went on to say that:

The part of the week will be a memorable one in the history of Heckmondwike from the singular fact that so extraordinary a number of deaths have taken place.[24]

The victims named included those from well-known local families, businessmen and trades people. Charles Burnley and his wife of Ings House within three days of each other, the latter on the day her husband was being buried. Charles Burnley was a trustee of Upper Independent Chapel and a member of the John Burnley and Company family and the coffin bearers were selected from heads of departments at the Grove Mills. Other well-known victims were Harry Liversedge, one of the most respected tradesmen in the town, and George Gledhill of Lobley Street, a talented violinist. The most 'painful case' was to be found on Dewsbury Moor where a man named King had lost his wife and daughter and was himself lying dangerously ill. The deaths had all been, readers were told, from one or other of the numerous chest infections accelerated by, or associated with, influenza. It was also clear that the deaths were not occurring solely amongst those who were living in the 'dwellings of the poor where there were many back-to-back cottages and overcrowding of persons'.[25]

The following week brought more bad news especially as it was reported that 'the number of interments at the Heckmondwike cemetery is a matter of common remark'.[26] This news was clearly supported by the clear evidence in the obituary column of the *Cleckheaton and Spen Valley Guardian*. The number of death notices had risen to eighty-four. The regular grave digger in Heckmondwike was laid up by the common enemy and the resources of the local undertakers were taxed beyond measure.[27]

Cruel Lives

Schools were now beginning to be affected and attendance was down right across the Spen Valley and the Heavy Woollen District*. At St. Luke's National School at Moorbottom, Cleckheaton, the headteacher recorded in the school log book that 'the influenza epidemic has just reached us. The average attendance is about twenty-five below foregoing weeks'.

This was, in fact, only the beginning, and in the weeks that followed some schools closed until the epidemic was over. This action was in some cases, perhaps, the result of staff absence. At St Luke's we read that on 25 May Miss Brayshaw was away with influenza. When the epidemic was over, the school was still noticing its after effects as a July log book entry indicates that members of the staff had had the delicate health of six children drawn to their attention.[28]

It was becoming clear during the second week of May that many of the attacks were now of exceptional severity and the fact that people had already suffered from the disease appeared, it was reported later by Robert Morrison, the Cleckheaton MOH, to offer no immunity.[29] This was, in fact, an issue that was raised in the *BMJ* in the autumn. Dr. Franklin Parsons, had asked at the annual conference of the British Medical Association for assistance from colleagues in answering the question: To what extent, if any, is one attack of influenza protection against another?[30] We now know, of course, that each wave of influenza is often of a

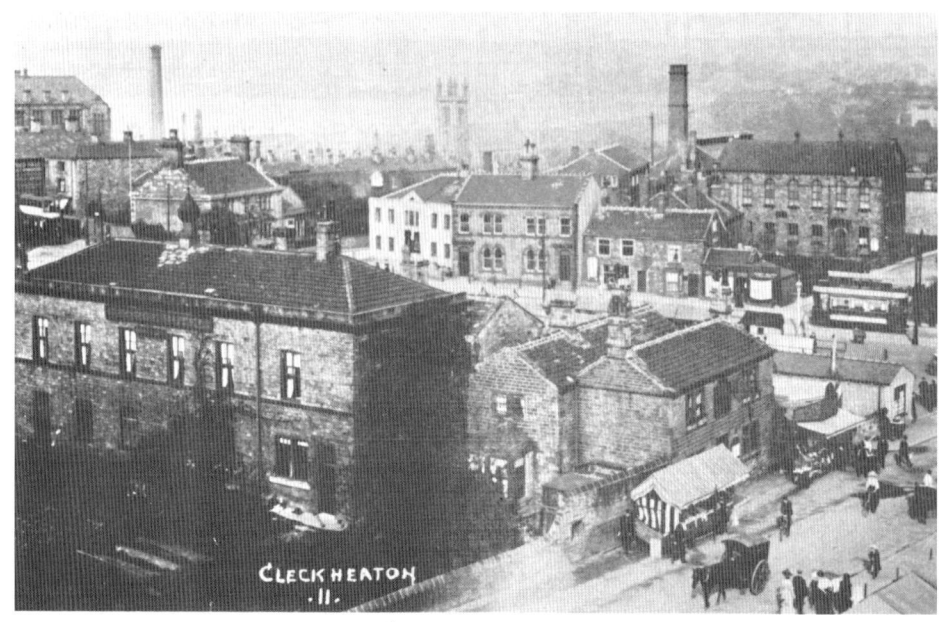

Figure 6:2 Cleckheaton in 1905.
(Margaret Wood: 'Cleckheaton in Times Past')

The tram (centre right) is travelling on Bradford Road. The Town Hall can be seen in the top left hand corner. The George Hotel is in the foreground.

---

*The Heavy Woollen District is named after the heavy cloth produced in its mills. Towns at the centre of the district are Dewsbury, Batley, Birstall and Heckmondwike, with Cleckheaton, Liversedge, Gomersal and Birkenshaw at its western edge.

different strain to the one previously experienced.

On 9 May the people of the Spen Valley and the Heavy Woollen District were informed that the area was receiving a 'severe and prolonged visitation' of that scourge, the Russian Influenza.[31] It was making inroads in families both rich and poor, as we have seen, and a fact that will become even clearer as we move through May. The state of affairs had become 'positively alarming'. Industry was being affected and a number of factories were shorthanded. At this stage children do appear, on the whole, to have escaped the disease although schools continued to close. Again, however, it was the staff who were being attacked with the virus, and at Boothroyd Lane Board school, for example, the school closure was the result of six staff being absent - perhaps 75 per cent of the teaching force.[32]

In Heckmondwike and Liversedge the disease was reported to be extremely prevalent and the appearance of the cemetery had changed considerably owing to the large number of new graves. There had been fifteen burials during the four days from Monday 4 May. This sight along with the many funeral cortéges passing through the town on a regular basis can have done little to encourage the local people. In Gomersal things appeared to be slightly better, where the MOH, Dr. Octavious Steele, had reported only one death by 9 May. Things were also 'better off' in Birkenshaw despite, the *Dewsbury Reporter* indicated, 'a large proportion of miners in the population'.[33]

By the following weekend the disease was reported, somewhat optimistically, to be on the wane. It had, however, already transported young and old to the 'house beyond the grave'. Readers who counted the deaths recorded on 15 May in the *Cleckheaton and Spen Valley Guardian* would have little doubt about this. The total was now ninety-three and would, the following week, peak at 101.(see table 6:1) It is perhaps important to recall here that eight weeks earlier, in March, the weekly figure had been thirty-two on the thirteenth and thirty on the twentieth. By 24 July the figure was down to seventeen.[34]

Table 6:1 Weekly death notices in the Cleckheaton and Spenborough Guardian: March-August 1891.

Week. ending	Death notices	Week ending	Death notices	Week ending	Death notices
6 March	41	1 May	57	3 July	17
13	32	8 *	84	10	35
20	30	15*	93	17	31
26 (Easter)	13	22*	101	24	17
3 April	61	29	57	31	23
10	46	5 June	39	7 August	18
17	44	12	46	14	16
24	34	19	29	21	21
		26	30	28	14

As can be seen the epidemic was at its most lethal during May, with 392 death notices, and especially during the middle three weeks* of the month.

We have already heard of the problems encountered in Heckmondwike cemetery, but Cleckheaton cemetery in Whitcliffe Road appears to have coped with the increase in interments. Other burials would, of course, have taken place in churchyards. These increased in May to 24, after figures of nine and twelve respectively in March and April. Burials recorded in June and July were again down to eleven and ten. [35]

The Victims

Details in relation to the victims were limited by the space available in the newspapers but the deaths of one or two 'public characters' continued to be reported in some detail. John Wood, a woollen draper and tailor of Wood View Cottage, George Street, who had a business in Westgate, Heckmondwike had died aged seventy-five. He had retired a few years earlier but continued to be busy in Sunday School life, as president of the local board, and 'other labours of a philanthropic kind'. He left a widow, Mary, five daughters and three sons. There is a most interesting side story attached to the life of John Wood. His grandson Arthur H. Wood, the son of John's son George, (see figure 6:3) born January 1875 in Heckmondwike, became a London theatre orchestra conductor and a composer. One of his compositions, *Barwick Green,* became the signature tune for the long running BBC radio series *The Archers.*[36] By 1891 the family had moved to Strawberry Dale Avenue, Harrogate and Arthur was by then a musical student and his father a music teacher and organist. When Arthur Wood died in January 1953 the *Spenborough Guardian* judged him to have been 'one of the most distinguished musicians produced from Yorkshire in the present generation'.[37]

Figure 6:3 1881 Census: King Street, Heckmondwike.

Name (All surnames Wood)	Relation to head of family	Condition as to marriage	Age	Occupation	Where born
George H	Head	Married	30	Tailor	Heckmondwike
Henrietta	Wife	Married	27		Mirfield
Arthur H.	Son	Single	6	Scholar	Heckmondwike
John	Son	"	4		"
Elizabeth J.	Daughter	"	2		"
Florence M.	Daughter	"	1month		"

Those suffering from the disease 'very severely' were Charles Fisher, the respected village postman in Roberttown and George Ackroyd a tailor and draper in Heckmondwike. They had both been 'badly used by the foul complaint'. At Clifton, a village just outside the Spen Valley, it was reported that James Dargue and his wife Margaret aged forty-six and forty-seven respectively, of Poplar Grove, had both succumbed to the scourge. James Dargue worked for the Low Moor Iron Company as an engine tenter and was a member of the highways board in the village.[38] Perhaps the saddest news came from Birkenshaw where a wool sorter, Alfred Speight, had committed suicide while, we read, temporarily insane from a severe attack of influenza.[39]

A Memorable Visitation

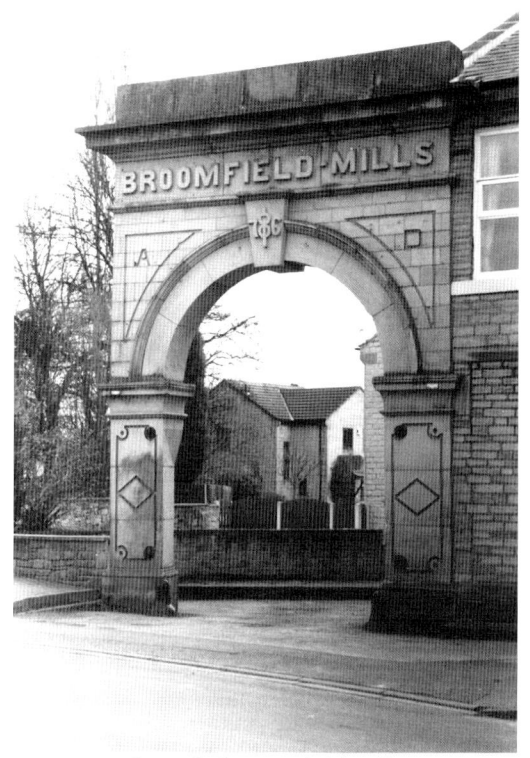

Figure 6: 4 Broomfield Mills.
The fine entrance archway is all that remains of the mills that were demolished in 1982[42]

Readers of the Spen Valley and Dewsbury papers learned on 22 and 23 May respectively of the deaths of more well-known local people. On the previous Sunday, Whitsuntide, Benjamin Craven, the caretaker at the Central Methodist Church and Brooke Street School in Cleckheaton had died 'under the most distressing circumstances' aged fifty-three.[40] The wife of John Holdsworth, manufacturer, had died two days later on Whit Tuesday, aged 59, after only a few days' illness. Two days later the 'dire scourge' took the life of mill-owner Elymas Wadsworth. His death not only shocked the town of Cleckheaton but also the hundreds who worked at the giant woollen spinning Broomfield Mills at Moorbottom.[41] Broomfield Mills were demolished in 1982 and nothing remains today except the fine entrance archway. Yet, as Barbara Wadsworth has indicated, 'the soul of Elymas's endeavour lives on in the vernacular of Cleckheaton'. Even today (2012) the site is still referred to as 'Waddies'.[43]

Elymas Wadsworth had been in poor health for some time but his death at the age of sixty-two had a profound effect on the town. He was a 'good man' and his death was deeply regretted.[44] He was also, clearly, very much involved in the life of the town and, at the time of his death, acted as chairman of the Town Hall building committee. He was also the principal benefactor. This was a considerable project for a local board with a population of, in Cleckheaton, 9,562; in Scholes 1,693 and Oakenshaw, 571. The imposing building, designed by Mawson and Hudson of Bradford, with its ninety by forty-five feet public hall and vaulted ceiling, is still used today as a public hall and council offices.[45] As Arthur Anderton, the vice-chairman of the building committee remarked at the time, the building has remained 'a monument that would

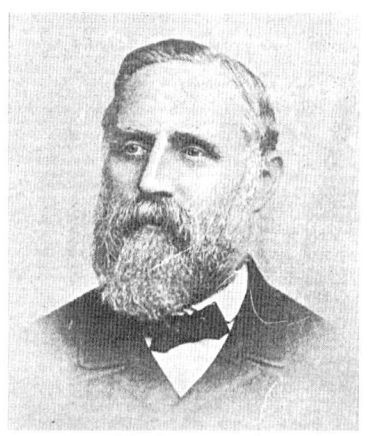

Figure 6:5 Elymas Wadsworth 1829-1891
(Frank Peel: Spen Valley Past and Present)

He never saw the Town Hall in its completed splendour [46]

Cruel Lives

stand for many generations'.[47] At the opening ceremony the following February, of the building Elymas never saw in its 'completed splendour', a memorial brass plaque in the town hall was unveiled in Elymas Wadsworth's name and later, in 1892, the clock was given in his memory by his family. The plaque notes that as chairman of the committee he gave 'willingly, largely and effectively of his time and substance'.[48] The Revd. E.W. Easton, vicar of St Luke's Church, the shadow of which fell across the Broomfield Mills, reminded readers of the parish magazine that the death of Mr. Wadsworth brought forcibly to mind, 'the slender thread by which our life hangs'.[49]

The funeral service took place, initially, at Broomfield House and the cortége then moved to Cleckheaton cemetery where the interment took place. Among the large number of mourners, in addition to Mr. Wadsworth's widow, five sons and three daughters, were many representatives of well-known influential local families such as the Burnhills, Laws, Mowats and Hirsts. They saw the ten oldest workers carry his coffin into the cemetery. Others in attendance were many of the 650 mill hands (Broomfield Mills closed for the day) and representatives of Providence and Westgate Congregational Churches in Cleckheaton. Elymas Wadsworth had worshipped at the former chapel prior to the opening of the one in Westgate, a project with which he was closely associated. Sergeant Lawson from the local police force and his constables were in attendance although, we read, their duties were merely onerous as the onlookers' behaviour was 'most decorous' throughout.[50]

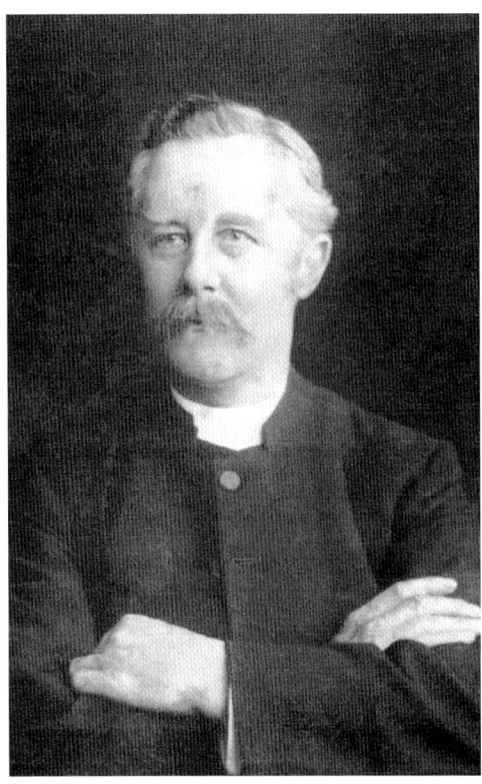

Figure 6:6 The Revd. E. W. Easton. Vicar of St. Luke's Church, Moorbottom 1885-1901
(The Story of a Church: St Luke's, Cleckheaton)

As in the case of Arthur Wood's grandfather there is also, remarkably, an interesting side story associated with Elymas Wadsworth, as Edward Wadsworth (1889-1949), the renowned artist, was his grandson.[51] Elymas's second surviving son, Fred, married Hannah Smith in 1888 and ten months later a son, Edward, was born in Cleckheaton. The family lived at Highfield House, Waltroyd Road off Westgate, less than three hundred yards from Broomfield Mills. However, within nine days of his birth Edward was left motherless, as Hannah died of puerperal fever. Edward, initially, grew up in the family home where his father was assisted by a nurse, a cook and a housemaid. From the age of ten he attended Godby's School (now Ghyll Royd) in Ilkley, as a boarder.[52]

A Memorable Visitation

Edward Wadsworth has been referred to as one of the most important artists of the first half of the twentieth century: a genius of Industrial England. As a student of the Slade School of Art he was a figurative painter but was, perhaps, most famous for his radically abstract work and his close association with Percy Wyndham Lewis (1882-1957) and the short lived vorticist movement.[53]

Wadsworth continued to visit West Yorkshire regularly after he had moved to London to study at the Slade in 1909.[54] He drew inspiration for a group of woodcuts when looking down from the hillsides, above the towns, on the industrial landscape of chimneys, factories and roofs. Figure 6:8 shows Cleckheaton, where the family worsted spinning mill was based. At first, suggests Jeremy Greenwood, the image

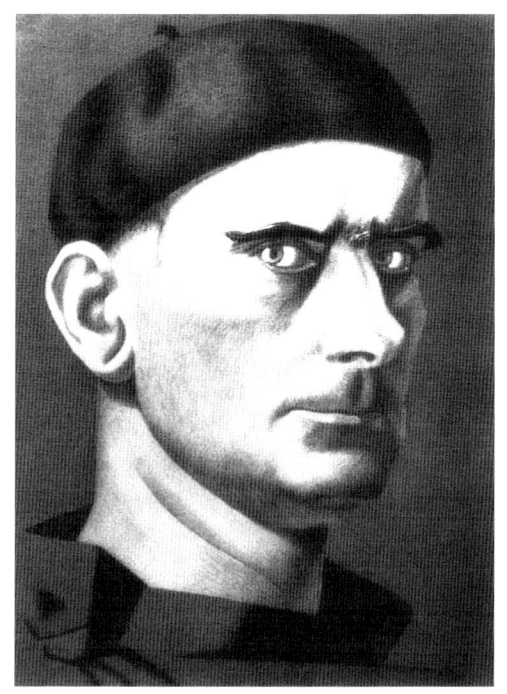

Figure 6:7 Edward Wadsworth: Self Portrait 1937
(The Estate of Edward Wadsworth)

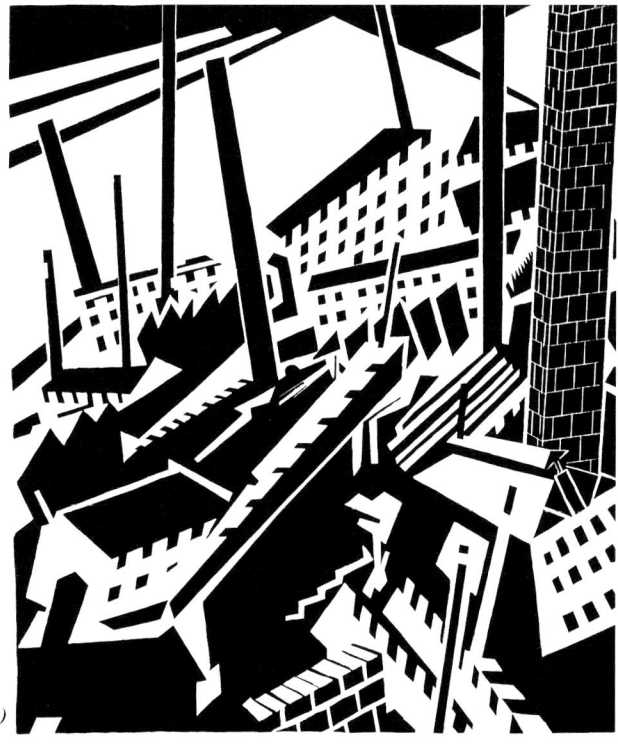

**Figure 6:8 Cleckheaton 1914.
An Edward Wadsworth woodcut.**
(The Estate of Edward Wadsworth)

appears to be entirely abstract but gradually a pattern of roofs and chimneys becomes apparent.[55]

On 29 May, just over a week after Elymas Wadsworth's death, there was little mention of the epidemic in the papers. By 12 June the epidemic was said to be over although its fire had been drawn by the end of May. However, deaths attributed to influenza continued to be reported. For example, on 12 June Mrs F. Ellis, a diligent worker for the Church Home for Waifs and Strays had died after pneumonia had set in. She had been attacked with influenza three weeks earlier. Deaths from pneumonia, bronchitis and other pulmonary afflictions were a recurring theme throughout the epidemic. As we shall see when the MOH reports are considered it is difficult to be precise about the number of deaths that were the direct result of the epidemic. Were, for example, the deaths of John Law, oatbread maker and newsagent, who suffered from bronchitis and to this his death was 'ascribed'; June Slack, the thirty-three years old wife of the Revd. George Slack, Congregational minister of Butts Villa, Westgate, Cleckheaton, and Dr. Campbell of Brighton Terrace, Heckmondike, who died on his twenty-eighth birthday, brought about by an attack of influenza?[56] The MOH for Huddersfield was clear about this when he identified the close relationship between influenza and diseases of the lungs. 82 per-cent of the victims' death certificates showed that the secondary cause of death was bronchitis or pneumonia.[57]

How many people did die as a result of the epidemic and what, when their reports were published for the year 1891-1892, did the medical officers have to say? A crude death figure can be obtained by considering the death notices in the papers when the epidemic was at its height with those at other times. The average weekly number of deaths announced in the *Cleckheaton and Spen Valley Guardian* for the six months March to August, excluding May, was 30.3. The weekly totals published during the five Fridays in May add up to 392. This shows an increase of 241 deaths compared with an average five weeks. Clearly not all these deaths occurred in the Spen Valley, nor on the other hand were newspaper notices printed for all the deaths that occurred, but the figure is significant.

Table 6:2 Age groups of victims.

Under one year: 41	31-40 years: 12
One-five years: 26	41-50 years: 16
Six-ten years: 2	51-60 years: 34
11-20 years: 4	61-70 years: 25
21-30 years: 11	71-80 years: 23

Numbers taken from death notices in the *Cleckheaton Guardian and Spen Valley News*: 15 and 22 May 1891.

The reports of the district's MOHs followed a similar pattern. As usual the reports covered a wide range of infectious diseases and suitable tables provided the necessary statistics. The reports, as ever, carried a commentary on the sanitary condition of the community for which they were responsible. For members of the local board, the comments must, in many cases, have made painful reading. Excrement disposal was a major issue and the River Spen or, as it often referred to locally, the 'Spen Beck' got worse very year and 'contained the usual quantity of sewage which frequently omits most offensive smells'. In Gomersal the water supply at the end of Great Gomersal was practically sewage and in Birkenshaw privy waste was sold to farmers and this was causing some concern.[58]

It was, however, the influenza epidemic that proved to be the focal point of most of the local reports. These were all published almost twelve months after the outbreak in the spring of 1892 but covered the previous year. The Liversedge report, handwritten by MOH John Shires, begins on a sombre note. Gentlemen, he writes:

Along with other districts in the country I have to put before you the most unfavourable report as regards the mortality which I have as yet made, there being upwards of one hundred deaths above the average of the past twelve years.

John Shires also drew the elected members' attention to the fact that the epidemic resulted in people succumbing not just to the prevailing epidemic of influenza but 'some of its sequilee'. This point was reiterated, as we shall see, by the Cleckheaton MOH in his report.

The number of deaths amongst the Liversedge population of 13,650 amounted to 342 giving a figure of 25.05 per thousand. The previous year's figures were 217 deaths (17.03 per 1000) eighty-one infants, many whose 'vitality was lowered by influenza and producing nervous disturbance' had died under the age of one year, and 130 under five years.[59]

Table 6:3 Liversedge Local Board

Year	1880	1881	1882	1883	1884	1885	1886	1887	1888	1889	1890	1891
No. of deaths	299	268	215	223	240	242	196	222	241	237	217	342
Rate per 1000	21.74	21.03	16.87	17.50	18.83	18.99	15.38	17.42	18.91	18.60	17.03	25.05

The annual death figures in Liversedge during the eleven years prior to the epidemic, and for 1891, provide a good example of the outbreak's effect on the death rate. The MOH also reported that 81 infants died under one year of age equal to 23.68% of total deaths, and a total of 130 died under the age of five. (38.01% of the total mortality).

In Gomersal Dr. Henry Octavious Steele, of Lane Side House, the district's MOH reported that although deaths from respiratory diseases had increased, the total number of deaths there, where the population was approximately four thousand, had been seventy-one, including thirty amongst those over sixty. This produced a figure of 17.75 deaths per thousand living.[60] In Birkenshaw members of the board received a similar report, from their MOH Dr. R. A. Forsyth, as there had only been a few cases of influenza amongst the population of 2,699.[61] The Gomersal and Birkenshaw news was in sharp contrast to that from Cleckheaton, the focal point of the Spen Valley. Many of the cases here, amongst the population of 9,562, had been of 'exceptional severity'. The death rate had risen from 16.84 per thousand in 1890 to 21.13 in 1891. The MOH Robert Morrison noted in his report that sixty-six deaths were the result of diseases of the chest, pleurisy, bronchitis and pneumonia, as many people had been weakened after suffering from one or more attacks of influenza.[62] Deaths from these causes was also the main factor in the phenomenal rise in the mortality rates during the influenza's prevalence in Bradford.[63]

These reports were written, as we have seen, almost twelve months after the outbreak. Even after considering them it is difficult to give a precise figure regarding the actual number of deaths in the Spen Valley that were caused by the influenza epidemic. Using as a guide an overall increase in deaths, as shown by the MOH reports, of approximately six per thousand of the population, the deaths directly related to influenza would be in the region of 240 as the population of Cleckheaton, Heckmondwike, Liversedge, Gomersal and Birkenshaw was approximately 41,000. This figure correlates with my original projection related to the death notices in the *Cleckheaton and Spen Valley Guardian*.

One thing, though, is certain. By the end of May the epidemic had reached its climax. Readers of the Cleckheaton newspaper would have been relieved to read that it was hoped by the end of July, an extremely cautious estimate, that 'this memorable visitation, which is said we owe to the filthy habits of the Russian people…will cease to cause anxiety'.[64]

In the light of recent fears relating to avian flu and the danger of a worldwide panic it is, perhaps, appropriate to end with the thoughts of A. H. (Arthur) Gale in 1959. No one, he said, can prophesy what the future of influenza will be, 'but the temptation to speculate is irresistible'.[65]

Chapter Seven

When Panic Seized the Town

The 1892 Brighouse Smallpox Epidemic

The Brighouse smallpox epidemic had its origins at a cottage near Vine House Farm in Savile Lane, Clifton during late April 1892, where Samuel Briggs and two of his children were found to be suffering from the disease. The infection quickly spread to the town and the first recorded case there, in early May, occurred at the home of Henry Child, a cab driver, in Daisy Croft.

New cases appeared in Brighouse at regular intervals throughout the summer months: in Rastrick, in Clifton and, to a lesser extent, in Hipperholme and Southowram. The epidemic struck great fear in the people of the district for although the community was used to epidemics such as measles and scarlet fever that also claimed lives, smallpox was a disease that was not only highly contagious and life threatening, but extremely frightening owing to its after effects such as pitting of the skin.

Brighouse became something of a ghost town as the epidemic raged, when people stayed away from the central shops and the more populated areas. Schools closed for lengthy periods and church attendance figures plummeted. Families affected by the disease were confined to their homes and this, along with a programme of vaccination and the hurried erection of an isolation hospital at Clifton, did much to contain the disease that at one stage was believed to be out of control.

The Nature of Smallpox

Smallpox, described in the first edition of *Pears Cyclopaedia* as the 'most loathsome of all the contagious diseases'[1] was arguably also one of the most dreaded during the years surrounding the Brighouse epidemic. It was highly infectious and spread through droplets of moisture produced when coughing or sneezing. When inhaled and absorbed by its victims, the microbe multiplies in the lymph glands. Other sources of infection included the handling of sufferers' clothing and bedding, where the virus could remain for a significant period of time, and the corpses of victims.[2] In fact only the decomposition or destruction of the corpse rendered it free from infection. These factors inevitably led to whole families being infected, especially those living in cramped and dismal conditions, where they often shared just one bedroom, with three of four siblings sometimes occupying one bed.[3] Smallpox, indicates F.B. Smith, was essentially but not always,

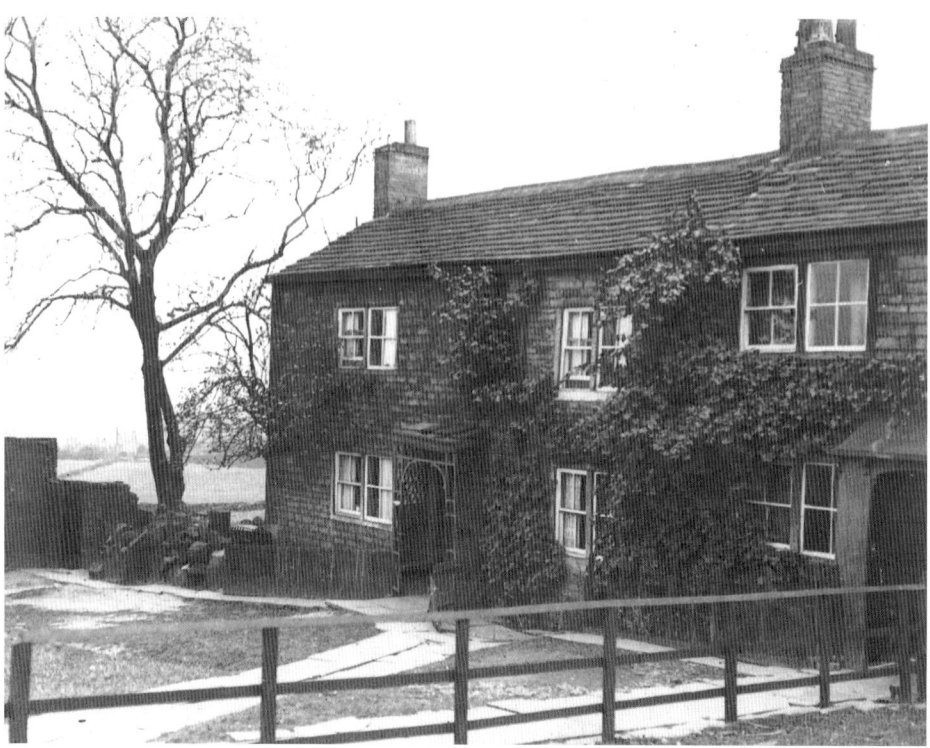

Figure 7: 1 Vine Farm, Savile Lane, Clifton in the 1950s
(Douglas Quarmby Collection)

It was at a cottage near Vine House farm, as the building was then known, that the epidemic began.

as we shall learn, a disease of the poor. It was also, notes Dorothy Crawford, a classic crowd disease and reached its peak during urbanization in the nineteenth century. Charles Dickens, among others, often highlighted the conditions of the poor and their illnesses; and it is generally assumed that the nameless fever that left the wonderful Esther in *Bleak House* scarred, after she nursed her sick maid, was smallpox.[4]

The people working and living together in camps, such as those occupied by the railway navvies and their families, were also particularly vulnerable. Outbreaks occurred at many sites, but one of the worst was at 'Batty Green' in 1871 during the building of the monumental Settle to Carlisle Railway when eighty died.[5] This outbreak resulted in the vicar of St Leonard's Church at Chapel-le-Dale writing to the Midland Railway asking for a subscription towards the cost of extending the burial ground. The company gave £20.[6]

Smallpox has a long history and epidemics of a disease that may have been smallpox were recorded in ancient Egypt and what is now Iraq, then Mesopotania, thousands of years before Anno Domini. The mummified remains of the pharaoh Rameses V who died in 1157 BC in his early thirties, and two other mummies, bear pustules indicative of the disease.[7] Before the appearance of syphilis (the great pox) in Europe at the end of the fifteenth century smallpox was known simply as pockes or pox. These terms being derived from the Anglo-Saxon *poc* for a bag or pouch.[8] Western Europe does appear to have been spared the virus that causes smallpox until around AD 1000 when it spread gradually until around the fifteenth century when it spread more rapidly.[9] By the seventeenth century it was very much part of British life. In 1710, for example, it was responsible for over three thousand deaths in London alone.[10] In 1871, 23,062 people died from the disease in England and Wales; the following year the figure was 19,022. In 1892, the year of the Brighouse outbreak, the national figure was down to 431. The number of deaths from smallpox declined rapidly after 1900, with the exception of 1902, and after 1906 passed fifty on only one occasion.[11]

The disease was at its most contagious during the first week but often continued to be highly infectious until all the scabs had dropped off. The 'most distressing premonitory' symptoms began with a rash that developed into pus filled blisters. Other symptoms often included high fever, fatigue, backache, vomiting, diarrhoea and a severe headache.[12] Misdiagnosis was not uncommon, as we shall see from the initial outbreak in Clifton, and even as recently as 1967 when there was an outbreak in South London, the first case was misdiagnosed as chicken pox.[13] People feared smallpox more than many other Victorian diseases. In addition to the inevitable fear of dying from the disease, those who recovered were often left with the tell tale pitted scars. In fact, one of the reasons people have always been so fearful of smallpox has been the disfigurement as much as the death rate. Those who did recover were often also left with bone infections, pneumonia and eye infections.

Smallpox respected neither age, nor wealth, nor beauty and throughout history killed, or seriously affected, many high profile figures including members of royal families. Queen Elizabeth I was badly scarred following an attack four years into her reign. Charles II's brother, the Duke of Gloucester and his sister Mary, the mother of William III, both died of the disease in 1660 aged twenty-nine and twenty-one respectively. Mary's husband had died from smallpox ten years earlier aged twenty-four. The future looked bright for the Stuart family in 1660 but within a generation smallpox had wiped them out following, amongst others, the death of Queen Anne's heir William (she had already lost two daughters to the disease) who died in 1700 aged eleven.[14] Away from royalty, those affected by the disease included Josiah Wedgwood, the founder of the pottery firm and grandfather of Charles Darwin, Joseph Stalin the Soviet dictator and John Metcalf the Yorkshire road builder. Metcalf became blind at the age of six following an attack of smallpox; Stalin was badly scarred by an attack and would often have his photographs retouched. Josiah Wedgwood contracted the disease in 1742 when aged eleven. It left him scarred and also with a knee joint badly affected. Eventually this became so badly disabled that surgery became inevitable. On 28 May 1768, his house-keeper wrote to staff that 'Mr. Wedgwood has this day had his leg taken off, and is as well as can be expected after such an execution'[15]

The work of Edward Jenner did much to control smallpox through vaccination following what he discovered from local farmers who believed that people did not catch smallpox if they had already had cowpox. He recorded that 'cowpox protects the human constitution from the infection of smallpox' and submitted his findings to the Royal Society for publication in 1798. There was, however, much opposition to his ideas although parliament supported his work with a £30,000 grant to open a clinic in London. He called the technique vaccination, named after the Vaccinia virus that causes cowpox and vacca, the Latin word for cow.[16] The vaccinia virus offers protection against smallpox as it shares, it is generally agreed, crucial molecular similarities with *variola major*, the deadly smallpox virus, that allow the human immune system to defeat the more dangerous agent. However, Dorothy Crawford has indicated that, in addition to those who support the cowpox link, there are those who also believe that smallpox is the human form of monkey pox. Further, and more recent studies, have even linked smallpox to camel pox and gerbil pox.[17] The *variola major* variety would more than likely have accounted for more than 90 per cent of the cases during the Brighouse epidemic.[18] We shall hear more of the work of Jenner, and others who introduced earlier methods of protection, as our story unfolds.

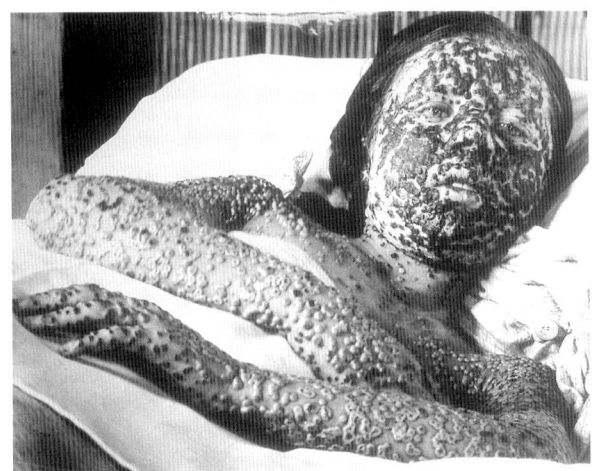

Figure 7: 2 A smallpox patient in 1923
(Copyright Dr. Jenner's House, UK)

The Brighouse Smallpox Epidemic Begins

Up until 1892 smallpox had only been a distant fear for many of the people of Brighouse, although there had been an outbreak of the disease in 1862 that claimed the lives of many young children. So when the *Brighouse Echo*, published on 6 May of that year, reported that there were two cases of smallpox at a house in Clifton the people of the district were not unduly worried.[19] They believed it was perhaps an isolated incident and Clifton was, after all, a separate community. Smallpox was not, though, just one of the most feared and life threatening diseases of Victorian Britain, it was also one of the most virulent. A week later the inevitable occurred and the disease reached the town. The Brighouse smallpox epidemic that was to affect the community for over a year had begun and within a short period of time panic had seized the town.

The initial outbreak in Clifton occurred in late April 1892 at the home of Samuel Briggs, a mason, who lived with his wife and four children in Savile Lane at a cottage near Vine House Farm. He had been suffering for some time from what was initially thought to be a skin disease, and was being nursed at home. However, when his two youngest children, James aged three and Sarah Ann aged one, were taken ill, a Dr. Carter of Rastrick was consulted and he pronounced the children to be suffering from a mild attack of smallpox. They had, he suggested, caught the

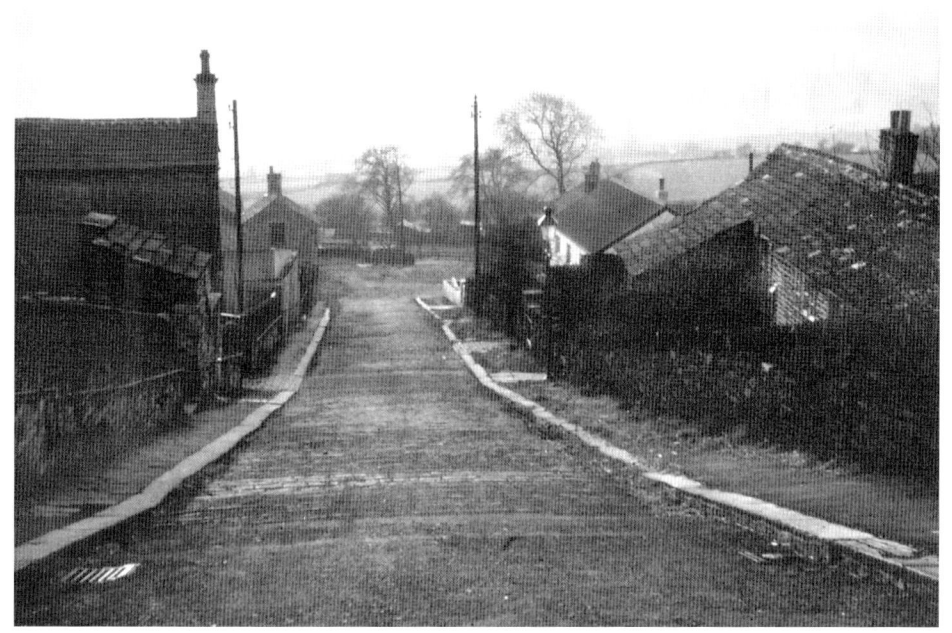

Figure 7:3 Savile Lane, Clifton in the 1950s.
(Douglas Quarmby collection)
Vine House Farm, the site of the initial outbreak, is situated at the bottom of this road.

disease from their father with whom, along with their mother, also called Sarah Ann, and two other siblings they shared what was probably the house's only bedroom.[20]

On the following Sunday, 1 May, the two infected children were removed to the Halifax fever hospital, at Stoney Royd, where they were reported to be making satisfactory progress. Their hospitalisation was not, however, before what Dr. Daniel Ainley, the Medical Officer of Health for the Halifax Rural Sanitary Authority, that embraced Clifton and Hipperholme, described as a 'great mischief' had been done. When he visited the house prior to the patients being removed to hospital he found that the mother had gone to a funeral in Brighouse and 'thus commenced a most serious outbreak'. An outbreak that we now know was the beginning of the 1892 Brighouse smallpox epidemic.[21]

The first cases in Brighouse occurred on Thursday 5 May, just after the *Brighouse Echo* edition that reported the initial outbreak in Clifton had gone to print, when it was discovered that the 'terrible and virulent disease' had broken out in Daisy Croft, and other cases quickly followed. Three members of the same family, Henry Child a cab driver, his son aged twenty-one and his daughter, aged fifteen, were found to be suffering from the deadly disease.[22] Soon the disease was to become virtually the sole topic of conversation in the ale-houses and shops as more and more homes were affected and death followed the 'frightening spread' of the disease.[23] On 13 May the *Brighouse Echo* reported that the disease seemed to have spread with 'astonishing rapidity' and that the cases were not confined to one part

Cruel Lives

of the town and went so far as to say that:

It is questionable whether in the past history of the immediate locality there has ever been experienced such a state of things as has transpired since the last issue of the Echo.[24]

The *Brighouse News* published a day later than the *Echo*, on Saturday, 7 May was already concerned that the 'malady' had assumed alarming proportions in the Clifton district, as several new cases had broken out in Savile Lane in close proximity to the Briggs's home. There was concern also that the Halifax authorities were 'disposed' to close their hospital in Halifax to patients from the out districts.[25]

The epidemic in the areas surrounding Brighouse began, perhaps, long before it was originally made public and Medical Officer of Health reports suggest that there had been reported cases as far back as January in Hartshead. In his report Dr. Ainley also records that in January 1892, the grandchild of the vicar, the Reverend Thomas King, who had been the incumbent since 1876,[26] was reported to be suffering from small pox at the vicarage. The child had been sent from Wakefield out of the way of his father who was suffering from the disease. The child died a few days after the initial diagnosis, in the Halifax smallpox hospital. The inmates of the vicarage were vaccinated and remained in quarantine for two weeks.[27] No further cases emerged in Hartshead until Tuesday 3 May when a young man by the

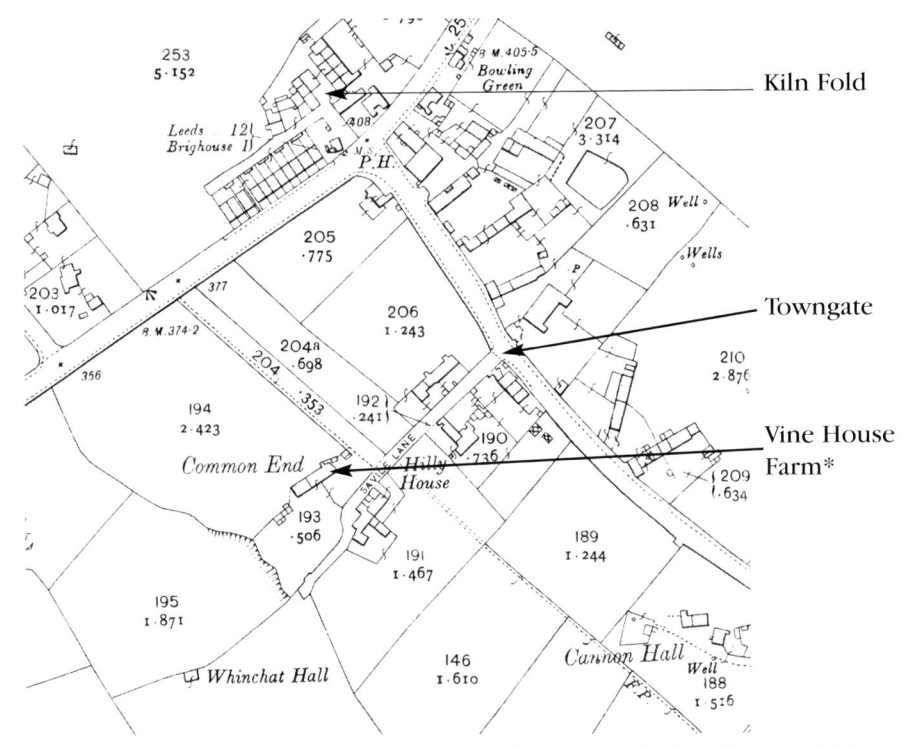

Figure 7:4 **The site of the initial outbreak in Savile Lane*, and Kiln fold where all the homes were infected**.
(Ordnance Survey 1907. surveyed 1892, revised 1905. Scale 1:2500)

name of Delaine, a collier, was removed to the Halifax hospital and the following Thursday George Oldfield of Littlethorpe, close to the first victim's home, was also taken to the same hospital.[28] The disease was also prevalent in Liversedge during the early part of the year and following a doctor's visit to that area he reported that he came across 'some very dirty houses inhabited by slatternly women whose husbands are colliers'![29]

The St. John's School, Clifton, log book certainly indicates that the disease was in the village before the date indicated in the *Brighouse Echo* as the Headteacher, John Tomlinson, recorded the following in the log book almost two weeks before the first case was reported in the papers:

25 April. (Monday) Opened the school. Smallpox has broken out in Savile Lane.[30]

How, we wonder, did he know this as the disease was not confirmed until the latter end of the week, and certainly after the Brighouse papers published on 29 and 30

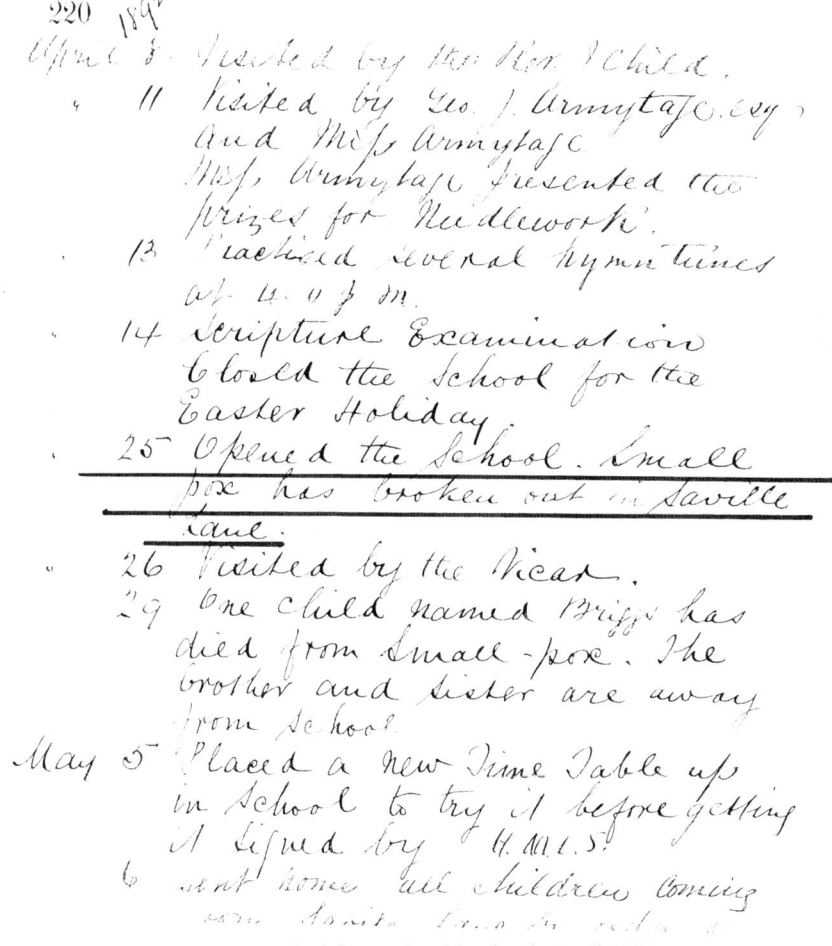

Figure 7:5 Clifton School log book, April 1892
(St. John's Primary School Clifton)

April had gone to print? Was the entry correct as a further entry four days later indicating that a 'child named Briggs' had died from smallpox is, according to our research, incorrect. Samuel Briggs had been ill for some time but a 'medical man' had seen him and pronounced that he was suffering from a skin disease. It was some time later, as we have heard, that smallpox was diagnosed. Perhaps the head's entry was based on the 'rumour being circulated' and the 'considerable excitement' created in the village.[31]

By 6 May all children living in Savile Lane had been sent home and the school closed the following day by order of the medical officer. It remained closed until 4 July. Just over a week later, on 13 July, the school was used as a polling station for the Parliamentary Election. The problems were far from over, however, as the head recorded only two days after the election that there had been several fresh cases of smallpox and understandably parents were again 'afraid of sending their children to school'.[32] John Tomlinson was headteacher at Clifton for thirty-four years, from January 1883 until April 1917 when he was succeeded by John Goring from Preston.[33] 1892 was a difficult year for the headteacher. He and the school managers, including the vicar, the Reverend John Child, who had become the first incumbent of the parish of Clifton when it was formed out of the Parish of Hartshead in 1887, would no doubt, have been pleased to receive an encouraging report from Her Majesty's Inspector at the end of the year. This indicated that 'under the circumstances the discipline and attainments are very satisfactory'.[34]

In addition to the new cases reported on 7 May in Clifton, in Brighouse a young man living in Clifton Road by the name of Sutcliffe, a collier, and John Taylor aged eleven of Firth Street, Rastrick, the son of a coach builder, also named John, were suffering from the disease. Sutcliffe was removed to the Halifax hospital but no further cases appeared likely to be admitted from Brighouse as the authorities did what they had been threatening to do and reserved the accommodation for those living in Halifax.[35] This decision prompted cries for an infectious diseases' hospital to be established in Brighouse. In fact, a public meeting was held at the Public Offices in Brighouse on 7 May at which a suggestion was made that a 'capital site' was available in Thornhills Road, Clifton on land belonging to Robert Ramsden, a farmer.[36] This, as we now know, was the site agreed upon and a temporary hospital was established there by 20 June. There had been similar calls for a fever hospital in Halifax in 1872 during a smallpox epidemic in that town, and an infectious diseases hospital had been quickly established in a former gentleman's mansion at Stoney Royd. Later, a separate smallpox hospital was built as it was found that a variety of diseases could not be treated satisfactorily under one roof.[37]

The disease appears to have spread rapidly and the cases were not confined to one part of the town although Police Street, Phoenix Street and King Street were initially the chief centres of infection. The areas affected during the second week included additionally, Back Bethel Street, Back New Street, Clifton Road, Brookfoot, Stack Garth in Ogden Lane and Daisy Croft. In Clifton seventeen outbreaks had been reported by 11 May and, in addition to Savile Lane, these were in Clifton Common, Kiln Fold, Towngate, Collier Row, at a farm in Grave Lane and

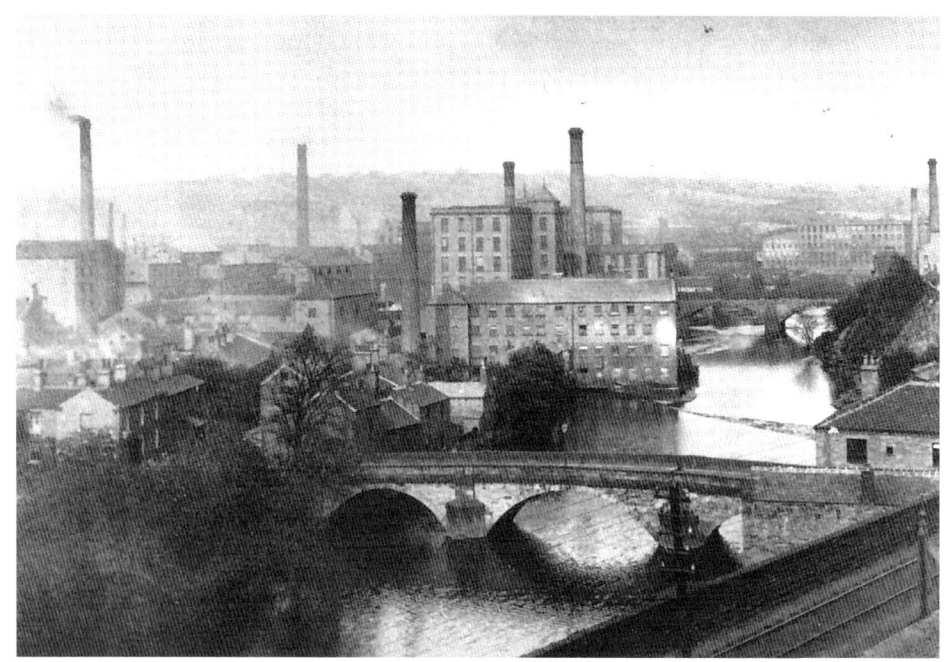

Figure 7:6 Brighouse in 1894.
(Chris Helme collection)
The town is seen here from the junction of Thornhill Road and Lillands Lane, Rastrick.

near the Old School Yard. In one house four cases were reported. At this stage the attacks were nearly all of a mild nature but a few cases were assuming more sinister characteristics owing to additional complications.[38]

Other areas surrounding Brighouse were also reporting cases. On 12 May the first case appeared in Hipperholme, at Thornhill Cottage, when the source of the infection was Halifax.[39] However, when a second person was diagnosed on 13 June the origin of this case was believed to be Brighouse. The two cases were treated in their own homes and 'strict measures' were adopted to prevent any further outbreaks. The Hipperholme district knew little at this time of the severe outbreak that was to gain a firm hold in November.[40] In July four cases of the disease occurred in Southowram, one of which was to prove fatal and again the source of the outbreak was traced to Brighouse. As with Hipperholme, more cases were to emerge as the year progressed.[41]

Inevitably, Brighouse became something of a ghost town with people too frightened to visit the usual town centre stores. Shopkeepers were clearly at risk, and on the 13 May it was reported that three assistants from the Co-operative central stores were absent suffering from the disease. Young people were also vulnerable. The school in Clifton, as we have seen, was closed until further notice and pupils from the Clifton area attending Brighouse schools were soon asked to stay at home. Pupils attending other schools in the district were also being kept at home by their parents.[42]

Cruel Lives

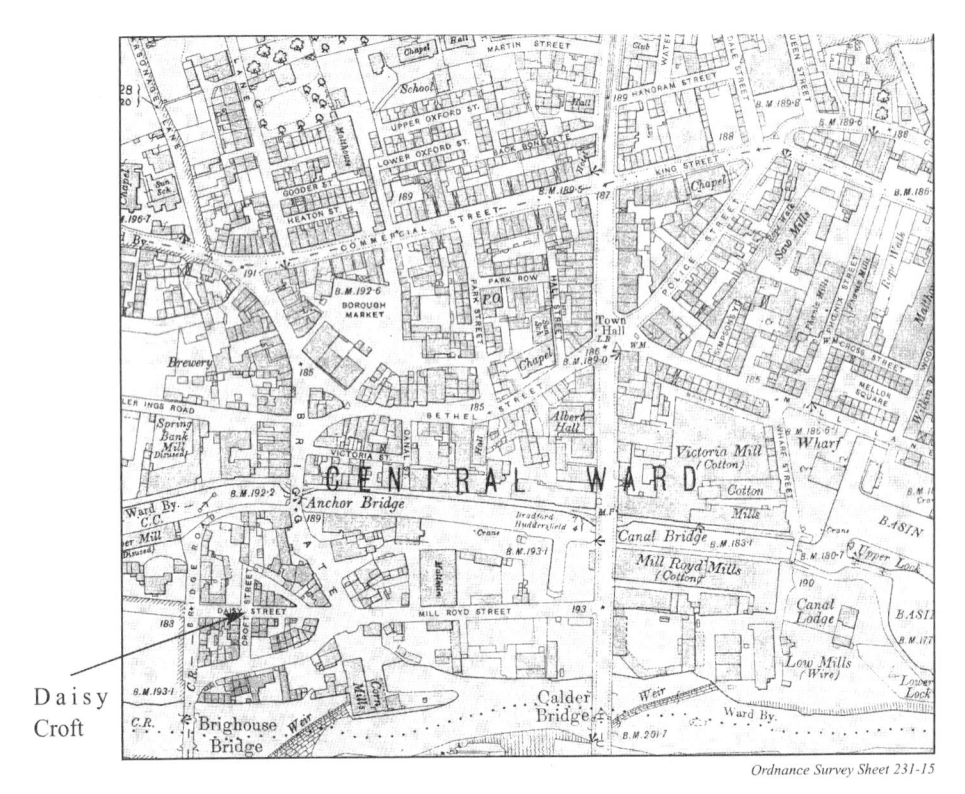

Figure 7:7 Brighouse town centre as surveyed in 1892.
(Ordnance survey map original scale 1:2500. Published 1907)
Daisy Croft was the site of the first outbreak in the town.

The head of Rastrick Common Boys School recorded on 27 May that 'the parents are afraid and keep the boys away' and the headteacher at the Church Infants' School in Rastrick recorded on 20 May that 'the parents seem to be keeping them away from fear rather than actual sickness'. At St. Martin's Girls' School in Brighouse the headteacher noted that several parents had visited the school to say, that once the examination was over, their children would not be attending until the smallpox disease had abated. The boys attending the Rastrick Common School from the Brighouse area had little choice in the matter, as they were sent home by the Medical Officer of Health on 20 May, and Rastrick Grammar School closed three days later. A similar situation arose in Brookfoot, and on the 16 May the headteacher recorded that as the disease was so prevalent in Clifton and Lane Head that pupils from those districts were being sent home. Sunday schools also closed and the May Whitsuntide treats were postponed indefinitely. Eventually, all the public elementary day schools in Brighouse were closed but the decision was, apparently, 'regarded by many as a questionable one'.[43] Despite the 'vigilance' of the mothers, the children were playing out in the streets and causing the same risk of infection. Other log book entries give us an idea of the way that the pupils' attendance was affected by the disease in their midst.[44]

6 May: Small-pox has broken out in the neighbourhood and Jno. R. Taylor is ordered to keep away from school, there being a case in his family. (Rastrick Common Boys' School)

20 May: Emily Stott is absent because of the death of her uncle caused by the epidemic. (Rastrick Church Infants' School)

24 June: Edgar Whitwam is away having a brother down in smallpox. He has been removed to the hospital which has been opened this week. (Rastrick Common Boys' School)

The First Deaths

The first deaths from the disease occurred on Friday 13 May when Illingworth Bottomley, aged four, the son of Taylor Bottomley a collier of Savile Lane, died. Later on the same day the death of John Taylor, aged eleven, of Firth Street was recorded. On the following Monday James Bickerdyke, aged thirty-four, a music and pianoforte dealer of King Street, and organist at Bridge End Congregational Chapel since 1885, passed away leaving a wife and three children. He had acquired a 'worthy reputation' in local musical circles and taught for a time at Rastrick Common School. He was buried in Rastrick cemetery.[45] Clearly the disease was not just affecting those living in the poorer areas of the town. On the following Wednesday, Elizabeth, the wife of James Beevers of Kiln Fold died aged forty-three. The interments in each case were 'effected as privately as possible'. In addition to these deaths there were now over fifty other cases of the disease in the district and that, according to the *Brighouse Echo*, the 'baneful and virulent scourge' of smallpox appeared to be spreading.[46]

Further cases came to light as the summer approached and it is likely that there were real fears amongst those in authority that things could get out of hand. The *Brighouse News* reported on 28 May that, 'it is with regret that we record the spread of the epidemic which prevails in our midst'. The death of Bridget Thrippleton, the wife of Albert a silk dresser of 10 Police Street (now Lawson Road), was a particularly sad case as she left eight children of whom the youngest, William, was eleven months old. William died in 1942 but his two sons were still living in the local area when the research for this section was carried out in 2002.[47] Bridget's death, aged thirty-six, was also associated with a tale concerning a pair of gloves. It appeared, 'if rumour be true',

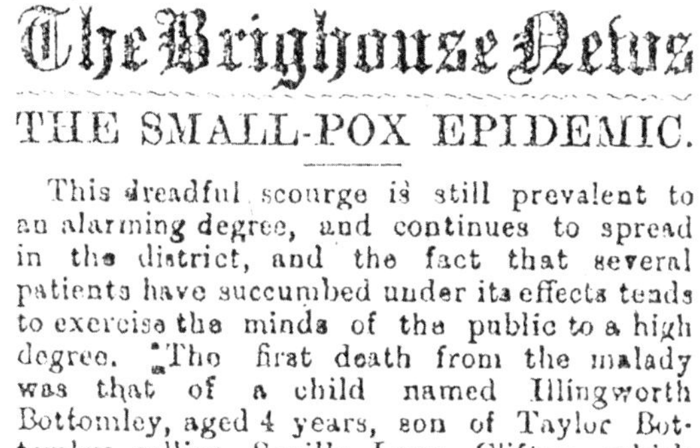

The Brighouse News

THE SMALL-POX EPIDEMIC.

This dreadful scourge is still prevalent to an alarming degree, and continues to spread in the district, and the fact that several patients have succumbed under its effects tends to exercise the minds of the public to a high degree. The first death from the malady was that of a child named Illingworth Bottomley, aged 4 years, son of Taylor Bottomley, collier, Saville Lane, Clifton, which took place yesterday evening week. Another death was notified during the evening, the victim being a son of Mr John Taylor, coach builder, Firth Street, Rastrick. On Monday evening Mr James Bickerdike, music and pianoforte dealer, King Street, Brighouse, succumbed to an attack of the disease, and on Wednesday evening the wife of James Beevers, collier, of Kiln Fold, Clifton, died from a similar cause. In each case the bodies were interred as privately as possible. The local

Figure 7:8 The Brighouse News, 21 May 1892
(Calderdale MBC Communities Directorate: Cultural Services)
The first deaths were reported in the local papers on Friday and Saturday 20-21 May.

that the victim lent a pair of gloves to a member of a family affected by the disease and it was therefore supposed that the gloves, when returned, were the cause of Mrs. Thrippleton's death. A similar case was reported in the Brighouse News on 21 May. Clothing had been sent out to wash from a home in Daisy Croft to a house in Police Street and in a few days the disease had made its appearance in the latter house. Rumour was, of course, always going to be a problem and 'considerable uneasiness' was being felt when reports that the disease had broken out in certain quarters, 'where such was not the case'. The victims of these rumours included a Mr. Denham of 75 Briggate, a cooper and dealer in fancy goods, and a Mrs. Newbold, a bread maker of Commercial Street.[48]

Figure 7:9 1891 Census Return, Police Street.

Name.	Relation to Head of Family	Age Last Birthday	Profession or Occupation	Where Born
Albert Thrippleton	Head	34	Silk Dresser	Brighouse
Bridget Thrippleton	Wife	36		Preston, Lancashire
Henry S Thrippleton	Son	15	Silk Dresser	Brighouse
Clara Thrippleton	Daughter	12	Silk Spinner	Brighouse
Laura Thrippleton	Daughter	10	Silk Spinner	Brighouse
Albert Thrippleton	Son	8	Scholar	Brighouse
Gertrude Thrippleton	Daughter	6	Scholar	Brighouse
Bertha Thrippleton	Daughter	4	Scholar	Brighouse
Nellie Thrippleton	Daughter	1		Brighouse

When Bridget Thrippleton died on 28 May 1892 she left eight children. The youngest, William, was not born when the census was taken.

The reporting of the outbreak in the local papers had been rational and honest. The story had been told in such a manner as to keep people informed without getting them unduly worried. However, during the week ending 4 June both the Brighouse papers decided that the outbreak was dying out. The *Brighouse Echo* indicated that 'there are signs of a distinct abatement in the smallpox epidemic' and the *Brighouse News* followed this by reporting with 'much pleasure' that the disease, with the exception of one portion of the township of Rastrick, appeared to be dying out. How they could be so optimistic is difficult to understand, as the same editions carried reports that a young man lay in a critical condition in Firth Street and that there were several other cases in the same neighbourhood. Another case had emerged in Well Lane, Clifton, where a joiner Jacob Roberts was infected. Apparently he had caught the disease whilst laying out the body of a victim of the epidemic. The register now showed that there had been 116 cases affecting fifty-four houses. Fifty patients had recovered and at this stage there had only been five deaths.[49] The following week, however, the *Brighouse Echo* reported the death of Jacob Roberts at the age of forty-seven. He was a widower and left a son Harry, a cabinet maker, aged twenty-three.

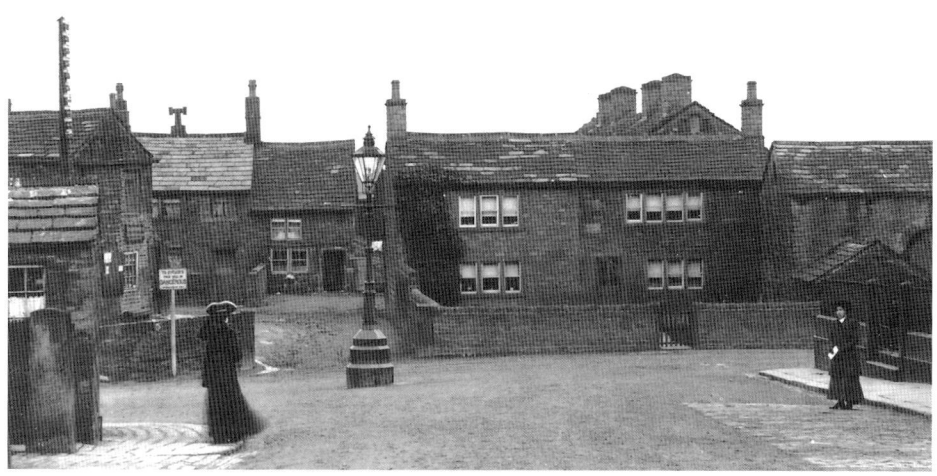

Figure 7:10 Kiln Fold Clifton c1904
(Chris Helme collection)

By 5 July 1892 every house in the fold was affected

Four weeks after the local papers' optimistic pronouncement, and following a period when only one death was recorded, that of Charles Wood on 21 June, a different story was being told. Charles, an orphan, whose mother had died of consumption two weeks earlier, was the first person to die in the Clifton Hospital that had only opened the day before his death.[50] We shall hear more of the hospital later, but twelve other people had been admitted to the hospital by 'closing time' on the hospital's first day, 20 June.[51] The *Brighouse Echo* found it 'unpleasant' to have to record that about a dozen new cases had been admitted to the hospital and new cases had occurred in Thornhill Briggs, Haigh Street, Park Street, Commercial Street and Queen Street.[52] In Clifton all the homes in Kiln Fold were now affected.

In almost all the new cases, the disease was of a 'somewhat severe and virulent' nature and on 15 July an 'astonishing escalation' in the number of deaths was reported. The first death of the week was that of the recently widowed Emily Redman, aged twenty-five, of Queen Street. Her husband Alfred, a silk spinning overlooker, had died of the disease on 3 June. The deaths of the young married couple afforded, noted the *Brighouse News*, 'one of the most pathetic incidents of the outbreak'. Others that followed included two children, Florence Smith and Barbara Scott, aged six and two respectively. The death toll in Brighouse was now twelve, yet the report concluded with the optimistic judgement that it was hoped that the disease was now dying out in the district![53] On 24 June the *Brighouse Echo* believed that it was 'still very gratifying to record a further diminuation' in the number of cases and a decline in the severity of the attacks. However, the same report also states that the epidemic in Clifton is very severe!

In Kiln Fold the disease still had the people in its grip and on 24 July it took the life of Eli Walton, aged twenty-eight. His death certificate is to hand and the cause of death, in addition to smallpox, was phthisis (consumption) and heart disease or, as it was reported, 'a complication of diseases'.[54] He died in the Brighouse and District Sanatorium [Clifton Hospital] where, encouragingly, it had already been reported, that the five nurses at the hospital led by Miss Roberts, the matron, were being 'assiduous in their attention to patients.'[55] Eli Walton left a widow, Florence, and three young daughters - Ann, Alice and Ada.[56] Four days earlier the deaths of Peter Clarke, aged two, of Back Bethel Street and of Lily Niblett, aged eighteen, of Southowram had been recorded. She was interred the following day 'at about midnight'. Lily's death, and Harry Farrand of Wyke's removal to North Bierley Hospital was, perhaps, an indication that the disease was now spreading beyond the town.[57] On 12 August the *Brighouse Echo* found it 'sad' to report another outbreak. At Waring Green a man named Mitchell was removed to hospital as were his four children. There were also outbreaks in Brook Street, Brick and Tile Terrace in Rastrick, and two more in Brighouse. On 20 August the deaths of one woman who resided at Hove Edge, and a child from Brighouse were reported - further examples that the disease still held the community in its lethal clutches.

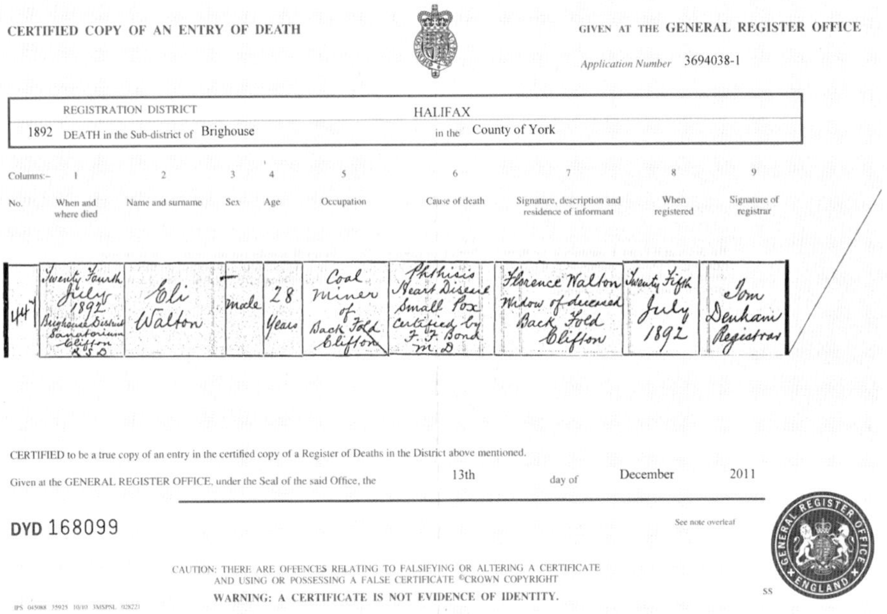

CERTIFIED COPY OF AN ENTRY OF DEATH

GIVEN AT THE GENERAL REGISTER OFFICE

Application Number 3694038-1

REGISTRATION DISTRICT HALIFAX

1892 DEATH in the Sub-district of Brighouse in the County of York

Columns:- 1	2	3	4	5	6	7	8	9
No. When and where died	Name and surname	Sex	Age	Occupation	Cause of death	Signature, description and residence of informant	When registered	Signature of registrar
447 Twenty Fourth July 1892 Brighouse District Sanatorium Clifton R.S.D.	Eli Walton	male	28 Years	Coal miner of Back Fold Clifton	Phthisis Heart Disease Small Pox Certified by F. F. Bond M.D.	Florence Walton Widow of deceased Back Fold Clifton	Twenty Fifth July 1892	Tom Denham Registrar

CERTIFIED to be a true copy of an entry in the certified copy of a Register of Deaths in the District above mentioned.

Given at the GENERAL REGISTER OFFICE, under the Seal of the said Office, the 13th day of December 2011

DYD 168099

See note overleaf

CAUTION: THERE ARE OFFENCES RELATING TO FALSIFYING OR ALTERING A CERTIFICATE AND USING OR POSSESSING A FALSE CERTIFICATE ©CROWN COPYRIGHT

WARNING: A CERTIFICATE IS NOT EVIDENCE OF IDENTITY.

SS

Figure 7:11 Eli Walton's death certificate.

(Home Office Passport and Identity service. Certified copy of an entry of death. Published courtesy of Mrs. Dorothy Holmes, Eli Walton's great grand daughter)

The following school log book extracts support the evidence that the epidemic was by no means over:

Rastrick Common Boys:

22-26 August. Tom Ematt and Robert Thornton are away through smallpox in the family.

2 Sept. Gough is now in the smallpox hospital.
16 Sept. Jas Watling is away on account of smallpox.
Clifton:
2 Sept. There have been several cases of small-pox.
11 Oct. Tom Payne's three children in school yesterday. The mother has been suffering from smallpox for 15 days.
21 Oct. Mr J Clayton's family next to the school-house have been removed to the smallpox hospital.

False Hopes

The ferocity of the epidemic did decline during the autumn and people began to feel that the disease was finally beginning to relax its stranglehold on the district. On 24 September the *Brighouse News* indicated that its readers would be glad to learn that no cases of smallpox had been reported in the Brighouse Local Board district for a period on a month. It was hoped that 'the dreaded disease had run its course'.[58] On 25 November only nine or ten cases were in hospital.[59] However, there were still set-backs and two deaths were recorded on 23 December: Those of James Hall Sykes, a young man from Bradford Road, and a young child in Thornhill Briggs.[60]

The worst was not over in Hipperholme, though, where the severity of the disease was still to be experienced as late as December. The doctors were not being helped either, as there were cases reported at the local board meetings where families had not informed the authority or Dr. Charteris, who was a member of the board, of smallpox cases in their houses.[61] Members recorded their 'disapprobation' of this fact. On 14 October it appeared in Lydgate, where there were eventually thirty-four cases. The local board called a special meeting on 17 October when it was agreed that:

The nuisance inspector be authorised to employ a sanitary messenger to attend to cases of smallpox in Lydgate, to supply them with food and prevent the inmates of the infected houses having any contact with the outside public. Permission granted to erect a temporary privy outside the Gelders' house for use of inmates.[62]

The disease continued to gain a foothold in Hipperholme and soon it had assumed epidemic proportions. Fifty-four cases were reported and forty-three of these were removed to the Clifton hospital.[63] The Lightcliffe National Schools (they were separate boys' and girls' schools at that time) were also closed for some weeks and vaccination or re-vaccination was offered to the residents of the district. These measures along with the disinfection and fumigation procedures that were resorted to 'with vigour' helped to control the disease.

In early December, the fear that the disease was spreading still further resulted in another Hipperholme Local Board emergency meeting, convened by telegraph, held at the Whitehall Inn. It was revealed at this meeting that their treasurer, John Sykes, had contracted the disease whilst attending to his duties.[64]

Cruel Lives

By the end of the year, however, there were signs that the outbreak in Hipperholme was on the wane and only one death was reported, that of man named Priestley who lived in the Lydgate area. The local board was pleased to receive the good news in relation to a decline in cases at their meeting on 13 December, but members were saddened to hear that their treasurer, John Sykes, was now confined to the hospital in Brighouse with the disease, and would be unable to present his usual collecting and deposit account.[65]

Church life was also affected with social activities continued to be cancelled. The Christmas services at St Matthew's Parish Church, Lightcliffe were badly affected with the church magazine reporting that the 'dreaded epidemic' had accounted for 'not a few empty places'. The number of communicants makes dismal reading as between 21 December and 22 January, a period that included nine mid-morning Sunday Eucharist services, a total of four celebrants (those taking communion) was recorded. 'A truly melancholy page in our church history' recorded the vicar, Alexander Harrison.[66] Was it though, he asked, entirely accounted for by the combined influence of the smallpox and the severe weather. Local sports fixtures were affected when three cricket matches involving the Brighouse Cricket Club were cancelled due to 'the raging epidemic'.[67]

There was, however, good news on the horizon. On 11 April 1893 Richard Dawson, the Hipperholme Medical Officer of Health was able to report that no cases had been seen since February, and he hoped that the district had seen the end of 'this unfortunate epidemic'.[68] In Southowram, around the same time, Dr. B.E.I. Edwards, the MOH for that local board, was reporting that since July of the previous year there had been eighteen cases, with six in one family, and three deaths, but in that district also there was cause for optimism.[69]

The last case in what was to become the newly created Borough of Brighouse and the surrounding districts, that was directly linked to the 1892 epidemic, was admitted to the Clifton hospital on 12 June 1893. It was the local boards that had handled the brunt of the disease and the new authority that brought together Brighouse and Rastrick on 9 November 1893. (Hipperholme, including Norwood Green and Coley, Southowram, and the Halifax Rural District Council, that included Clifton, carried on as separate bodies until 1937 when they were all, with the exception of a section of Southowram that was linked with Halifax, incorporated into the Borough.) There were, inevitably, minor outbreaks of the disease over the years and something of a mini-epidemic in 1902 when a lodging house in the town was at the centre of the infection. In November of that year eleven people were admitted to the hospital in Clifton suffering from the disease and two of them died. That particular outbreak continued until March 1903 and a total of five deaths were recorded. From that time until 1904, when the small pox hospital at Warley was used, the Brighouse small pox cases were sent to Hollins Hey Isolation Hospital at Elland. The Clifton hospital was now, as recommended some ten years earlier, a general infectious disease isolation hospital for cases other than smallpox.[70]

Table 7:1 Cases and deaths in the wider Brighouse area covered by this study-1892-93

	Cases	Deaths
Brighouse	134	15
Rastrick	40	5
Clifton	60?	2
Hipperholme	56	1
Southowram	18	3

Prevention

Residents in all the infected houses, as we have seen from the cases in Hipperholme, were requested to stay indoors and to absent themselves from work, although the employers were asked to pay their wages. In a number of cases the heads of families stayed away from their own homes, rather than risk losing permanently their 'daily avocations'. A case was reported concerning an engine tenter who had made his sleeping quarters in the engine room. Not everyone, it appears, conformed to the guidelines. When the Brighouse Health Committee met on 10 May it was reported by J.J. Lane that 'persons from infected houses were walking about the district' including a man whose wife was in a very dangerous state. 'Such reckless conduct', he believed, ought not to be allowed.[71] In August T. Shaw, a grocer of Park Street, had received a summons under the Infectious Diseases Notification Act, 1889 for failing to report two cases of small pox in his house. His daughter Annie had the disease and another daughter Clara had had the

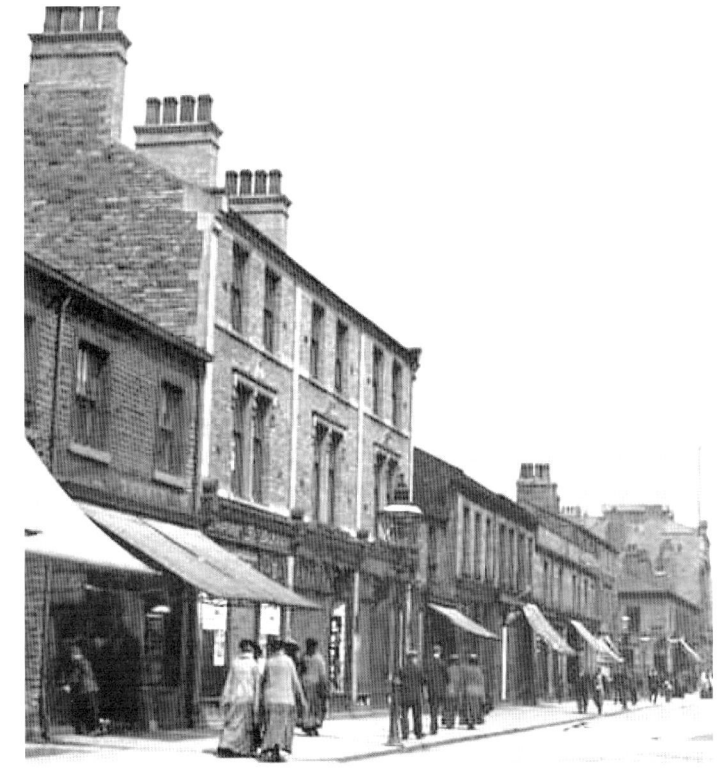

Figure 7:12
Commercial Street
Brighouse c1900
(Chris Helme collection)

During the height of the epidemic the town's shopping centre was almost deserted.

disease and was now convalescent, but was playing with other children in the street.[72]

People were employed by the local boards to convey groceries and other household 'necessaries' to the homes affected. In Clifton the role was fulfilled by John Dickinson aged seventy-three of Savile Lane, a gas lamp lighter. He had been appointed as the 'medium of communication' between the infected homes and the outside world. He visited each home several times a day with milk and groceries.[73] Did he and others, I wonder, knock on the door and run away after collecting the money that was, perhaps, left on the doorstep? Was money actually handled as even this was believed to be a risk? Readers who recall the 1962 outbreak in West Yorkshire, and especially in Bradford, may remember coins being placed in a bucket of disinfectant in some shops prior to being handled by the shopkeeper.

It is difficult to imagine just what life was like in homes where someone was infected. Consider what life was like for the Taylor family of Firth Street where a youth was infected and eleven other people were confined to the house.[74] Homes such as this were, however, visited by one or more of the four trained nurses who were working with the smallpox guru, Dr. Bond, who had been appointed Medical Officer of Health for the district, in charge of smallpox cases. The Vicar of Brighouse, the Reverend R.P. Steadman, also made visits to those who wished to see him. Requests were also made for parcels of linen, books, and toys to be handed in at public offices for delivery to homes affected by the outbreak.[75]

Figure 7:13 1891 Census Return, Firth Street.

Name.	Relation to Head of Family	Age Last Birthday	Profession or Occupation	Where Born
John Taylor	Head	44	Coach Builder	Devizes, Wiltshire
Mary W Taylor	Wife	42		Devizes, Wiltshire
Catherine Taylor	Daughter	16	Silk Operative	Huddersfield, Yorks
Ernest Taylor	Son	14	Silk Operative	Huddersfield, Yorks.
Albert G Taylor	Son	12	Errand Boy	Rastrick, Yorks.
John R Taylor	Son	10	Scholar	Rastrick, Yorks.
Ellen Taylor	Daughter	7	Scholar	Rastrick, Yorks.
Harry Taylor	Son	6	Scholar	Rastrick, Yorks.
Emily Taylor	Daughter	4	Scholar	Rastrick, Yorks.
Frank Taylor	Son	2		Rastrick, Yorks
George Taylor	Son	1		Rastrick, Yorks
Arthur Taylor	Son	2 months		Rastrick, Yorks

The 1891 census return gives details of the late Taylor family, who were incarcerated in their cramped house when John aged ten contracted the disease and subsequently died.

As soon as the epidemic took a firm grip on the community the local boards did all in their powers to prevent the spread of the disease. The isolation of infected people was one of the key forms of prevention. The other chief measures included the use of disinfectants and vaccination. At Rastrick Common Boys' School the head teacher used his initiative and decided to order carbolic soap for the boys to wash in and carboline in liquid form for the floors. The residents of the district were reminded to be watchful and diligent through the posting of hand-bills and notices. A general notice was produced for the area (see figure 7:14) but in Clifton the local people were specifically reminded not to make use of Savile Lane.[76]

Disinfectant was quickly made available to all who applied for it but the authorities found it difficult to cope with the initial demand. On Tuesday 10 May, the Brighouse gas works was besieged by requests and the supply exhausted within two hours. Chemists shops were also bombarded and one store sold out of camphor. In Clifton disinfectants were made available from Harry Bairstow in Clifton Common and from Charles Ramsden at the Armytage Arms, following the delivery of a cab full of supplies. It was also reported, on 13 May, that the 'vigorous and energetic' measures taken to prevent the spread of the disease included flushing the drains in the infected areas.[77]

Figure 7:14 Public notice in the *Brighouse Echo* 13 May 1892

> PUBLIC NOTICE – SMALLPOX.
> The above disease having broken out in the neighbourhood, the public are particularly requested to co-operate with the Sanitary Authority in checking the spread as far as possible.
>   1.- Do not go where it is on any account.
>   2.- If you have been near the infected places or persons be re-vaccinated at once
>   3.- Hold no communication by letter or conversation with any person living in any infected house or neighbourhood.
>   4.- All children and other persons unvaccinated should lose no time in applying to the public vaccinator.
>   5.- If you are taken ill with headache and sickness, and backache, send for the doctor at once, that he may tell you what steps to take.

However, whilst people were happy to use disinfectants they were less sure about vaccination. The residents of Brighouse were offered vaccination against the disease but many declined through lack of understanding and a fear that being vaccinated would lead to them contracting the disease from the effects of impure vaccine. The vaccination programme was in the hands of Dr. Bond the medical officer to the Rastrick Board who had been appointed, as previously indicated, medical officer in charge of small pox cases during the epidemic and later hospital superintendent. His appointment had the support of the Halifax Rural Sanitary Authority that embraced Clifton, Norland, Hipperholme and Hartshead districts, as well of that of the Brighouse and Rastrick Boards. He quickly established vaccination stations at Hartshead, Clifton and Brighouse and also vaccinated from house to house in areas of infection. Dr. Bond, members of the public were informed, was working indefatigably on behalf of the patients. A vaccination committee was also established with H.J. Turner of Brighouse as chairman and notices were posted in relation to vaccination and re-vaccination.[78]

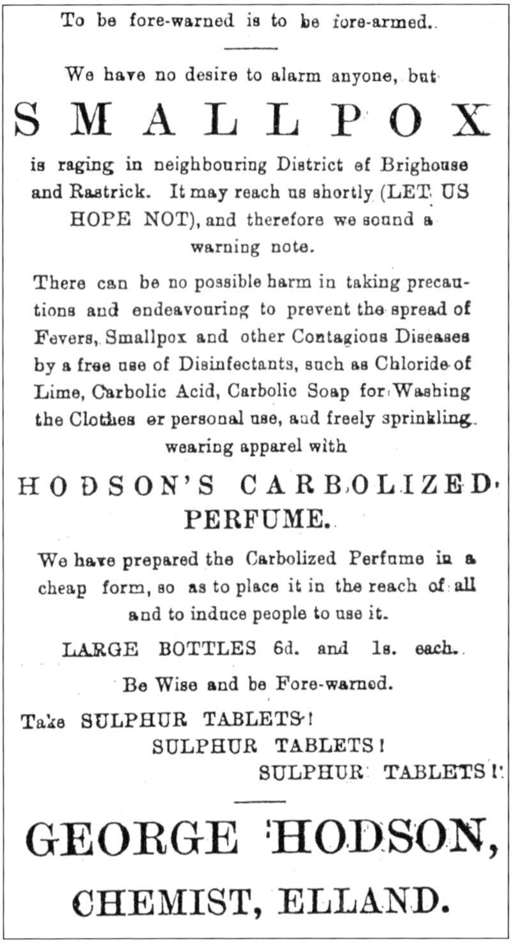

The 1892 vaccination programme, and the controversy surrounding it, was recalled in 2003 by Miss Isobel Sutcliffe. She remembered well how her aunt, Elizabeth Baldwin, the sister of her mother Annie, was apparently affected by the vaccine she received as an infant and died aged twenty-one. The family lived in Woodhead Lane, Clifton and her aunt was believed to be developing normally, both physically and mentally, until she was vaccinated.[79]

Despite all the publicity and the fact that vaccination, following Edward Jenner's discovery almost 100 years earlier, had reduced the death rate from smallpox enormously many people continued to be unconvinced.

Figure 7:15 Advertisement in the *Brighouse Echo* 3 June 1892.

This was one of the many products that purported to give protection against the disease.

Local doctors spent considerable amounts of their time offering advice to the general public as the following report makes clear:

In many cases I spent an hour or more setting the pros and cons of the matter before the people. Only in a few cases did I fail to effect it by moral suasion and argument.[80]

Edward Jenner, a Gloucestershire doctor, the son of the Reverend Stephen Jenner, was born in Berkeley, Gloucestershire, on 17 May 1749. Whilst an apprentice at Sodbury he listened eagerly to farmers and to a young countrywoman who indicated that she 'could not take' smallpox because she had had cowpox. He therefore began to set out to show that cowpox protected against smallpox and also that cowpox could be transmitted from one human to another as smallpox could. This is not the place for a full analysis of the medical and clinical background to Jenner's thoughts and work. However, his courage and determination took him into unknown territory on 14 May 1796. History was indeed made on that day.

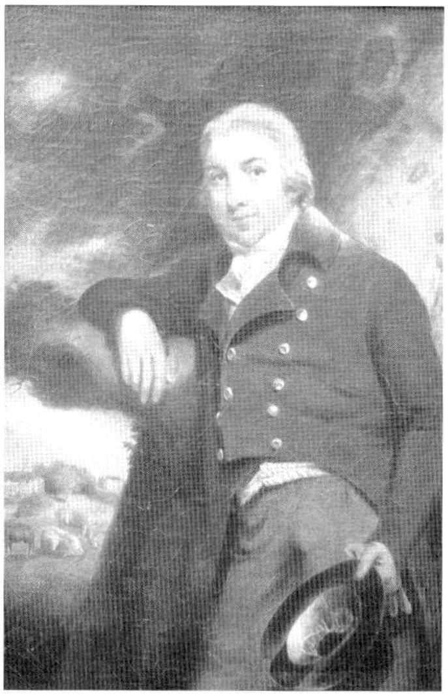

Two weeks earlier Jenner had found that a dairymaid, Sarah Nelmes, had a typical cowpox lesion on her finger. He then used matter from that lesion to inoculate eight years old James Phipps with cowpox. On 1 July Jenner then inoculated in both upper arms the boy with matter from a smallpox pustule. After many long days and nights Jenner noted that no smallpox symptoms resulted and he immediately submitted a paper to the Royal Society. Other experiments followed, and in 1798 he vaccinated John Baker, aged five, with material from an infected cow and recorded seventeen other cases of people who appeared to have obtained immunity from smallpox after contracting cowpox directly from cows.

Figure 7:16 Edward Jenner (1749-1823)
(Copyright Dr. Jenner's House, UK)

Jenner was, then, the discoverer of vaccination and many support the view that 'few discoveries in science or medicine have had the impact to equal that of Edward Jenner'. He also had time to take a deep interest in the natural world around him. In 1788, he presented a paper to an initially disbelieving Royal Society on his research related to the cuckoo. He showed how a day old bird ejects all its foster siblings from the nest and is then reared by its foster parents, who believe the cuckoo to be their own.[81] This modest man died following a stroke in 1823 and is buried in Berkeley.[82]

Prior to Jenner's work, the traveller Lady Mary Montagu Wortley had introduced inoculation here from Turkey. As a young woman she had been greatly admired for her beauty but an attack of smallpox in 1715 when she was twenty-six left her disfigured. She had also lost a brother to the disease. The practice that she observed whilst in Turkey involved the insertion of a small amount of matter from a pustule of a patient with a mild form of the disease, into the skin of a healthy person.[83] She described in a letter to a friend how smallpox parties were held. At these peasant women would perform inoculations. Her letter did, though, include the quite frightening description of how an 'old woman comes with a nutshell full of the matter…she immediately rips open what veins you please to have opened'. This, in most cases, caused only a mild attack of smallpox. The practice gained a powerful endorsement in 1722 when the Prince of Wales's daughters were inoculated. Many did, however, question the effectiveness and safety of inoculation. It is true that although some did die after undergoing the process, numbers were few in comparison to those who died after contracting the disease naturally. It was only a partial solution to the problem and smallpox continued to exact a huge toll across the world.[84]

Cruel Lives

The Brighouse and District pro-vaccination group received a welcome boost on 29 May 1892 when the Reverend George Hill gave an address at the Methodist Church in Rastrick that received wide publicity in the local press. He asked people to act upon the advice that they had received, including that given by the *Brighouse Echo*. His son was a doctor and advice to him from that source included re-vaccination, plenty of fresh air (he did not mention that this was in short supply in some parts of the town!), good exercise, good food and the avoidance of contact with patients. Dr. Bond was, he concluded, a man to be admired and he prayed that he would be brought safely through.[85] Clearly the vaccination programme also had the support of some members of the teaching profession, as the head of Rastrick Infants' School recorded the following in the school log book on 2 June:

I was absent on Tuesday and Wednesday morning because of my arm being very bad from vaccination.[86]

The vaccination controversy continued to rage and six years later, in 1898, the anti-vaccination group received a further, though indirect, boost when the Vaccination Act of 1898 was passed. This ruled that children should be vaccinated within a period of six months following their birth but allowed parents to receive an exemption certificate if they made a conscientious objection![87]

The following figures issued in the Brighouse Medical Officer of Health's report for 1892 make a convincing post epidemic argument for vaccination and support the efforts made by the pro-vaccination group. In the Brighouse Board area alone there were, as previously indicated, 134 cases of smallpox resulting in fifteen deaths. The details in relation to age groups affected and those vaccinated and unvaccinated are as follows:

Table 7:2 Brighouse Local Board-1892. Ages groups of victims and survival rates in relation to vaccinated and unvaccinated cases.[88]

Age profile of death	1-5yrs (5 deaths), 5-15 (2), 15-25 (1), 25-65 (7)
Vaccinated cases	103 resulting in 6 deaths
Unvaccinated cases	24 resulting in 9 deaths
Re-vaccinated cases	7 with no deaths

The death rate amongst those contracting the disease was, it was pointed out, over six times greater amongst the unvaccinated members of the population. The figures being 37.5 per cent compared with only 5.82 per cent amongst those who had been vaccinated.[89] The figures also show clearly that it was still possible for those vaccinated to be infected with the microbe, especially if the vaccination had taken place three to five years previously when the immunity was decreasing.[90] It is, however, clear from the case figures that a majority of the people had been vaccinated. Unfortunately similar information is not available for the Rastrick, Hipperholme, Hove Edge, Clifton and Southowram areas.

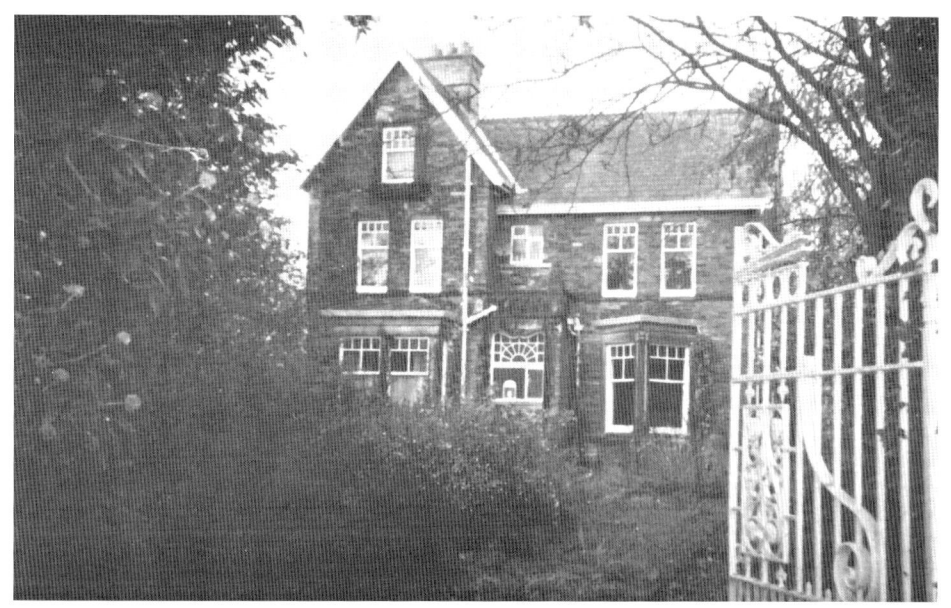

Figure 7:17 Clifton Hospital

The hospital's administrative block that included nurses' accommodation, in 2002. This building opened in 1897

The Clifton Hospital.

There were calls for an infectious diseases hospital to be established in the area almost as soon as the smallpox epidemic came to the notice of the community, and public feeling was running high. Everyone in the town, observed Mitchell, seemed 'possessed with incarcerating victims as soon as possible'.[91]

Four years earlier the West Riding County Council had received a negative response from the Brighouse Local Board to their suggestion that steps should be taken to provide an isolation hospital in the Brighouse area. This time the board did respond and at a meeting held on 6 May it was agreed to address the issue concerning a local hospital by asking the Rastrick Local Board, and the Halifax Rural Authority that represented Clifton and Hartshead, to co-operate in a joint venture.[92]

On Saturday 7 May, three members of the joint authority inspected land above Lillands Wood, Rastrick and mill premises, house and barn at Barker Royd, Southowram. Neither site was deemed to be suitable. At the meeting held on the same evening at the Public Offices in Brighouse it was agreed that five acres of land off Thornhills Road, Clifton, belonging to a farmer Robert Ramsden, should be considered on a seven year lease at £25 a year. There was an option to purchase the land at £150 per acre at any period that the committee decided. The site was inspected and terms agreed on the following day. It was decided, initially, to purchase an iron hospital in, we assume, kit form. On Monday 9 May members travelled to Liverpool to inspect buildings of that nature that were made there and to view the Liverpool infectious diseases hospital. It was, however, agreed that owing to the urgency of the situation, the building should be built on site by local joiners who would construct an inner shell of wood. This was to be covered with corrugated iron plates, produced by a Liverpool firm, similar to those used in the construction of iron churches. The building was to be 125 feet in length and, as the plan shows, would accommodate forty-eight patients.[93]

Workmen were quickly rushed to the site and Thomas Bottomley was appointed in charge of building work with instructions to seek the aid of other joiners. Many other local tradesmen were recruited including, for example, G. H. Firth of Rastrick who erected the brick foundations and J. F. Brown and company who provided the iron bedsteads.[94] A 'vigorous start' was made on 12 May. A matron and four nurses had already been employed by the time the work began and on the following day an advertisement for a cook was placed in the *Brighouse Echo*.[95] When a reporter from the paper called at the site during the following week he found the place 'veritably alive' with workers and that the framework of the main building was already in place. A large quantity of iron had arrived from Liverpool and workmen from that city were working on the roof. Amazingly the reporter concluded with the observation that some people, but not those 'who speak with authority', considered that the work had been too slow![96]

The reporter, it appears, was not the only one to visit the site as a vast number of visitors from all parts of the district had taken the opportunity to see the building work hoping, no doubt, that they would not be future residents. By the 28 May the press were able to indicate that it was hoped that the hospital would be ready to receive its first patients in two weeks.[97] This view was supported the following week when a representative from the *Brighouse Echo* found that the building was already assuming a finished look and that patients were likely to be admitted during the following week.[98] The rival paper, the *Brighouse News*, published a day later, had the advantage on this occasion. It was able to inform its readers that the hospital would be 'thrown open' to inspection by the general public on the following Saturday, 11 June, and patients would be admitted during the week that followed.[99]

On the day before, the premises had been inspected by medical officers, local board officers and fifty 'gentlemen.' Numerous expressions of surprise and delight were heard at the 'beautiful and elevated' position.[100] The hospital, as we have heard, admitted its first patients, thirteen in all, on Monday evening 20 June. The ambulance began its rounds once, we learn, the workmen had completed their finishing touches.[101] By 1 July forty of the forty-eight beds were occupied. It was not long, however, before the number of beds provided proved to be inadequate. Three large tents, two for sleeping and one for day use, had to be erected on wooden platforms. These were delivered to the station at Brighouse on 6 July from Norfolk. The previous Saturday W. Pilling, chairman of the committee, and the local board clerk, James Parkinson, had been 'despatched by train' to Norfolk to negotiate such a supply with an army contractor in Downham Market. On 15 July there were fifty-four patients in the hospital and 10 of them were in a critical condition.[102]

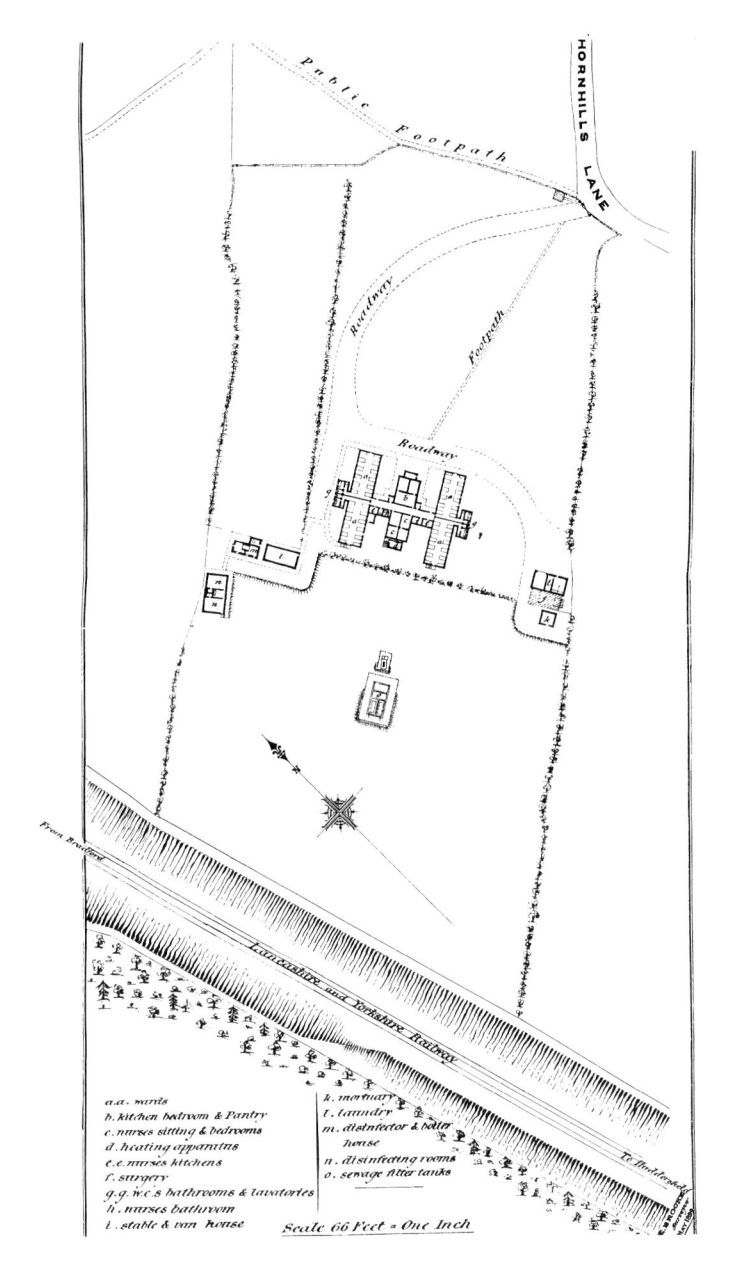

Figure 7:18 Clifton Hospital Site Plan May 1892
(West Yorkshire Archives, Wakefield. (Ref WRD7/6/1/35)

It was hoped that when eventually the area was free from smallpox that the building would be extended so as to accommodate and isolate those with other infectious diseases. The last case of smallpox left the hospital in June, 1893 and the premises were then left in the hands of the caretaker and his wife who had instructions to keep them in good order and ready for immediate use at any time.[103]

The hospital had cost £5020 2s 6d and this was apportioned amongst the authorities according to their population. When the Brighouse Joint Hospital Board was established in 1894 members decided at their first meeting on 6 April to seek a loan from the Local Government Board. Seven hundred and fifty pounds was requested for the purchase of the site, repayable over fifty years, and a loan was also sought to cover the cost of the buildings repayable over thirty years. The request, however, met with a mixed response. Money was available for the purchase of the site but not if it was to be used for the isolation of smallpox patients. This decision was made in Whitehall after:

Having regard to the relation of the site to the dwellings around it, upwards of 7,000 persons residing within a radius of half a mile from its centre, and in view of the accumulating evidence of the danger of smallpox spreading from a hospital in such a situation.

The site was considered to be well suited for the purposes of a hospital and a loan of £750 would be sanctioned, but only on the understanding that 'smallpox shall in no circumstances be received in it'.

£2,818 was also to be loaned against the buildings, a figure just over half that requested, owing to their temporary nature and the many shortcomings identified by architects. The main building was defective in both arrangement and construction, the wards were too narrow, inefficiently ventilated and warmed, and not provided with satisfactory closet accommodation. The floor space was only suitable for twenty beds.[104] Clearly the local Hospital Board had some thinking to do and some important decisions to make regarding the future use of the Thornhills Road site!

A decision was eventually made following a Brighouse Corporation conference on 5 February 1895, led by three doctors. The doctors supported the views previously conveyed to the local hospital board and based their recommendations also on what they had seen in Sheffield, Fulham and Bradford. It was agreed that the site should be used only for the treatment of general infectious diseases.[105] New buildings were constructed two years later at a cost of £5,000 pounds and the matron, Lily Waddington, was appointed at a salary of £50 a year. This was not quite the cottage hospital that many in the town had hoped for but it was a fine building that, although divided into flats, still stands today.[106]

Despite the problems related to life in towns in Victorian Britain, already highlighted, Brighouse did escape virtually all of the major outbreaks associated with the period. There was typhus in Rastrick in 1858 and an outbreak of cholera in 1862 but these did not compare with the heavy toll that these diseases, and others, exerted on other communities. The 1892 smallpox outbreak had made people very frightened but also thankful that the death toll was 'only' twenty-six. (ten more, however, than in the whole of England two years earlier). This figure has, of course to be put into perspective and compared with extrapolated figures for a larger town. Using the Brighouse Local Board area as an example the death rate was, when rounded, 1.5 per thousand (fifteen of the 10,500 population). Had the population been the size of, say, a city of four-hundred thousand the toll would have been six hundred!

The Brighouse district was not alone in suffering an attack of smallpox in 1892/1893. Halifax recorded 513 cases with forty-four deaths and in the Holme Valley there was a real sense of panic when cases occurred in New Mill, where some people 'fled from the place', and in Holmfirth.[107] The death toll from the disease nationally was declining as we have seen, and locally there were no more serious outbreaks. World wide this was not always the case but eventually Jenner's work was rewarded in the best possible way when the total eradication of smallpox was officially certified in Geneva on 10 December 1979.[108] The last person to die of the disease in the United Kingdom had been a Mrs. Janet Parker in September 1978. She who worked at the Birmingham Medical School, as a photographic technician, but how she was infected remains a mystery.[109]

Appendix

Key dates relating to the epidemic

25 April, 1892	Clifton school headteacher records in the school log book that smallpox has broken out in Savile Lane, Clifton.
1 May	James and Sarah Briggs of Clifton are removed to the Halifax smallpox hospital.
5 May	First cases of the disease in Brighouse, at Daisy Croft. More patients from Clifton are admitted to the hospital in Halifax
6 May	The *Brighouse Echo* reports an outbreak of smallpox in Clifton. This is the first public reporting of a case related to the epidemic.
7 May	Clifton school is closed indefinitely. Public meeting held in Brighouse in relation to hospital provision in the town.
11 May	Seventeen cases of the disease reported in Clifton.
12 May	The first case in Hipperholme during the current epidemic is recorded.
13 May	The *Brighouse Echo* reports that the disease has spread with 'astonishing rapidity'. First deaths recorded. Those of Illingworth Bottomley in Savile Lane, Clifton, and John Taylor of Firth Street, Rastrick
16 May	The organist at Bridge End Chapel, James Bickerdyke, dies from the disease, aged thirty-four.
28 May	Bridget, the wife of Albert Thrippleton, silk dresser of Police Street, dies aged thirty-six, and leaves eight children.

12 June	A twenty-five year old widow Emily Redman dies ten days after her husband Alfred.
20 June	Clifton hospital opens and admits its first patients.
21 June	The hospital's first death is recorded; that of Charles Wood, aged two years.
1 July	The *Brighouse Echo* reports that 12 new cases have been admitted to hospital.
5 July	An 'astonishing escalation' in the number of deaths is reported. All homes in Kiln Fold, Clifton are infected.
14 October	The disease appears again, in Hipperholme. The Lydgate area is badly affected.
12 June 1893	The last case directly linked to the epidemic is admitted to the Clifton hospital.

Brighouse smallpox epidemic deaths: May-July 1892

13 May: Illingworth Bottomley (4) son of Taylor Bottomley, a collier of Savile Lane, Clifton.
13 May: John Taylor (11) son of John Taylor a coach builder of Firth Street
16 May: James Bickerdike (34) Music dealer of King Street.
18 May: Elizabeth Beevers (43) wife of James Beevers a collier of Kiln Fold, Clifton.
25 May: Bridget Thrippleton (36) wife of Albert a silk dresser of Police Street.
5 June: Jacob Roberts (47) a joiner of Towngate, Clifton.
21 June: Charles Wood (3) an orphan of Park Street
3 July: Alfred Redman (25)* a silk spinning overlooker of Queen Street.
12 July: Emily Redman (25)* wife of the above.
13 July: Florence Isabel Smith (6)* the daughter of Henry Smith of Haigh Street.
13 July: Barbara Stott (2)* daughter of Albert a blacksmith of Back Bethel Street.
24 July: Eli Walton (28)* a collier of Back Fold, Clifton
29 July: 14 deaths had occurred by this date (Brighouse Echo)
The information available relating to later deaths is somewhat vague.
*Died in the Brighouse and District Sanatorium (Clifton Hospital)

This chapter has drawn heavily on the author's previous work *When Panic Seized the Town: The 1892 Brighouse Smallpox Epidemic.* Published in 2003 by Rastrick High School and written in association with sixth-form pupils Gemma Newsome and Katie Normanton.

Chapter Eight

A Baffling Outbreak

Diphtheria in Bradford, 1904

If we simply use Lawrence Sawchuk's definition of an epidemic as a guide, the diphtheria outbreak in Bradford in 1904 may not fall within our terms of reference. He basically defined an epidemic as 'a marked rise in the frequency of a specific infectious disease in a community over a limited period'[1] The Bradford outbreak was, then, no ordinary epidemic but is still worthy, for our purposes, of epidemic status. Indeed, as the Bradford MOH, Dr. Arnold Evans stated in his report to members of the council in 1905, diphtheria 'existed in epidemic form during the latter half of 1904'. There had, he indicated, been a 'phenomenal rise' in cases. He had already drawn the members' attention to the epidemic the previous November when he issued an interim report that began with the ominous sentence 'I beg to report the continued prevalence of diphtheria'. It had, in fact, begun to take on epidemic proportions at the beginning of the year with schools in West Bowling being closed 'owing to diphtheria' as early as 29 January.[2] At Woodroyd School Boys' Department the headteacher recorded on 8 February that:

Attendance very thin this morning. I think this is partly attributable to the several cases of diphtheria being in this neighbourhood, and other parts of West Bowling.[3]

Diphtheria was, along with measles, whooping cough and scarlet fever one of the major childhood diseases of the time. It was first clinically recognised in England during the 1850s and from 1856 was no longer classed with scarlet fever in the Registrar-General's returns.[4] Its history is in fact, according to Greenwood, 'intrinisically confused' with that of scarlet fever.[5] The disease caused great alarm amongst the British public when first identified although it was generally far less widespread than the other childhood diseases. The public alarm was, suggests Hardy, caused in part by the perception of the disease as new but also by the fact that it struck at random and the symptoms were highly distressing. Like scarlet fever it was not simply a disease of the poor and it had the distressing habit of descending on small and close communities and inflicting severe losses. It was, especially, a disease of households, schools and institutions.[6]

The modern history of the disease appears to have begun with what Gale refers to as 'the wave of prevalence' around 1855. In that and the following year, epidemics ascribed to diphtheria had been recorded in Launceston, Spalding, Billericay, Thame, and Ash in Kent. In 1859, 9,587 deaths were directly attributed to the

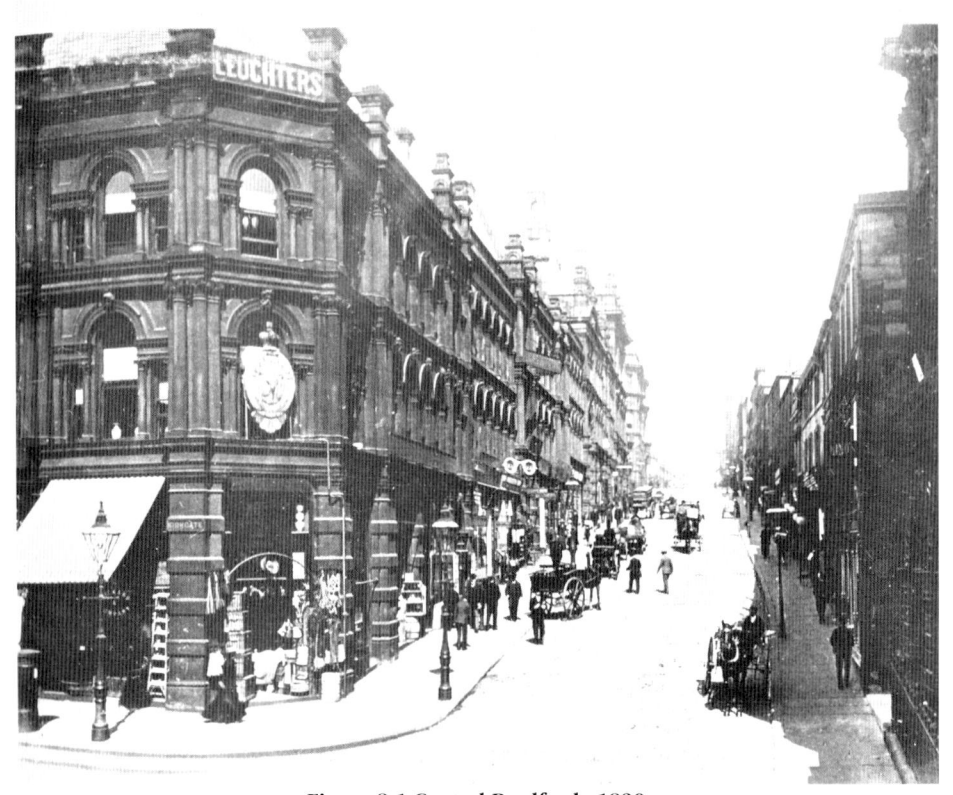

Figure 8:1 Central Bradford c1890
(Bradford City Council: Museums and Galleries)
This image shows Darley Street looking from Kirkgate. Little would have changed here by the time of the diphtheria epidemic in 1906.

disease and the victims were spread throughout England and Wales.[7] Between 1855 and 1869 diphtheria had been recorded as being responsible for sixty-one thousand deaths in England and Wales. About half the deaths were of children under five and of the remainder around 80 per cent were aged from five to thirteen. However, with what Smith calls uncertainty of diagnosis in mind, these figures should be accepted only as a guide. In fact every ailment of the throat was, according to Dr. Robert Semple, 'recorded as diphtheria'.[8] For example, the designation of most cases of diphtheria in Camelford in Cornwall during a severe four-year epidemic, as croup, was just one example of how the most experienced doctors had been lured into a sense of false security.[9]

The disease is caused by the organism *Corynebacterium diptheriae* and is spread by droplet infection, close contact, infected dust and contaminated milk. It developed rapidly from a sore throat into something more sinister. The growth of a whitish grey membrane over the back of the throat that, when linked with swelling, stopped swallowing or breathing, was the most widely recognised characteristic of the disease. This often required a tracheotomy that was performed when time was vital, records Wohl, with a hatpin or penknife.[10] The operation was also performed on serious cases in hospitals, once they began to admit diphtheria cases in 1888, but was only successful in a quarter of these.[11] In fact most general hospitals were reluctant to admit diphtheria patients. It was, however, the toxin and the highly poisonous state of the victims' blood that caused the deaths of so many. Those who recovered were often left with severely damaged heart or nerves.[12] As with scarlet fever the percentage of those contracting the disease who died was high and Wohl quotes figures of around 20-25 per cent.[13] The situation did improve somewhat after the bacterium was isolated and more especially after an anti-toxin was made available for general use in 1894. Before then doctors could not cope with the disease and were offered little in the way of so called cures. These appear to have chiefly taken the form of calomel and mercury preparations, sedation and isolation.[14] The eventual disappearance of diphtheria as a serious threat to the lives of children did not occur, suggests Hardy, until the immunisation campaigns that began after 1923.[15]

The reported incidence of the disease often baffled the authorities. It was worse in winter, more deadly in poorer houses, but it hit the comfortable too. The pattern of the spread of the disease in, for example, London during the period 1888-95, followed no set path. The disease appeared in every district during this time although some districts suffered more than others. Deaths in the poorer districts were above average possibly, suggests Hardy, due to poor resistance or delays in sending for the doctor, therefore delaying treatment.[16] However, three of the better off districts also suffered higher than average mortality rates and this resulted in the sanitary authority's wildly inaccurate theory that ventilators on the sewers were to blame. In fact the miasmic link between unhygienic sanitary conditions and diphtheria had proved 'enduringly popular' both with the general public and the sanitary reformers. As Smith indicates, the disease does not appear only to be related to industrialisation or slums.[17] Its lethal qualities do, however, seem to be linked to poverty and overcrowding.

Considerable Alarm

Prior to the year that is the basis of this chapter, Bradford appears to have almost entirely escaped any epidemic of diphtheria during the years when other areas were affected or, according to Newsholme in his *Origin and Spread of Pandemic Diphtheria*, in any other year. Leeds, for example, had suffered a moderate epidemic in 1883-84, Halifax a 'greater' one in 1886 and Huddersfield a much more severe one in 1887. In Bradford fourteen people did die from the disease in 1878 but the mean for the years 1871-96 was just seven.[18] This, as we shall see, was not the case during the 1904 epidemic[19]

In many ways this was an unusual epidemic and, as indicated, did not fall into the usual category of outbreaks of infectious diseases. It was long, in that it lasted at least a year; it did not follow a strong seasonal pattern, although it was more prevalent in October and, unusually, it did not attract a high level of publicity. In fact, the outbreak is hardly mentioned in the local papers. One of the few reports that I could find appeared as late as October 1904 when the *Bradford Daily Telegraph* reported that:

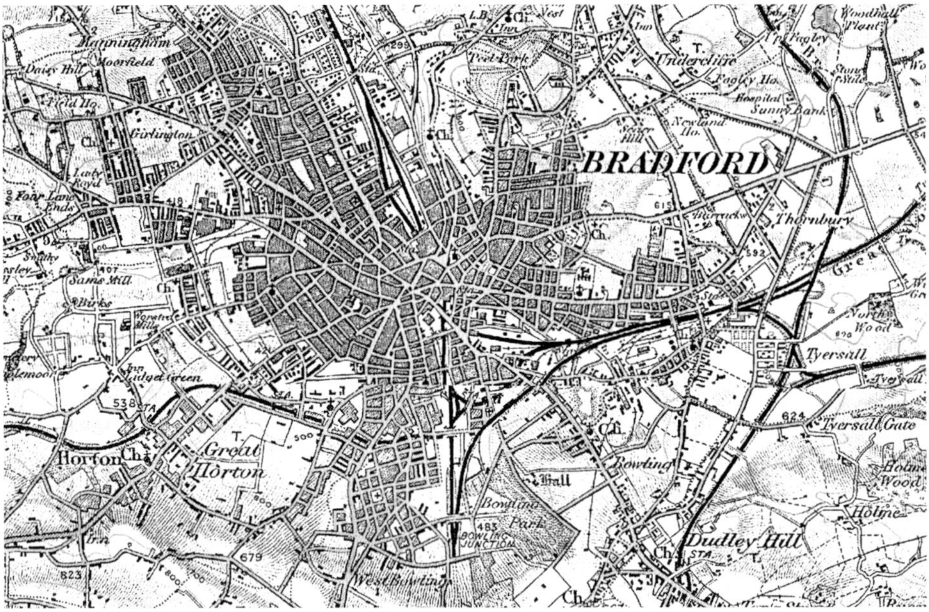

Figure 8:2 Bradford around 1900. The West Bowling, and Great and Little Horton areas were the most severely affected by the outbreak.
(Cassini Historical Map. Revised New Series, sheet 104. Original scale 1:50,000)

Considerable alarm is being felt by the sanitary authorities in Bradford at the rapid increase in scarlet fever and diphtheria in various parts of the city. The Leeds Road Hospital is crowded out and a new pavilion adjoining erected. The authorities are at a loss to explain the outbreak.

The majority of the hospital cases were at this stage suffering from scarlet fever and on 1 October there were 110 patients with the disease, five with typhoid, and 19 suffering from diphtheria. One death had been recorded, that of a diphtheria patient. Overall, however, 421 diphtheria cases were admitted to the Leeds Road Hospital and six to North Bierley. Schools closed at this time were, again, in West Bowling and now, following the scarlet fever outbreak, at Eccleshill and Idle. Others were to be closed in 'contemplation'.[20]

As we have heard, diphtheria was, like measles and scarlet fever, essentially a disease of childhood. These diseases, coupled with the desperate living conditions in the industrial towns, were the key factors in the high rates of infant and childhood mortality. High rates of infant mortality were, as Barbara Thompson has indicated, one of the most intransigent of all public health problems of the nineteenth century. By the 1870s Bradford, a town that had grown from a population of thirteen hundred people in 1801 to 180,000 eighty years later, had already acquired an unenviable reputation as a town with a high infant mortality rate. Many districts were grossly overcrowded and sanitary engineering was of a limited nature. The endemic disease in the town in the decades around 1860-70 was typhoid. It was not surprising then that mortality rates generally, and those of infants especially, correlated closely with the housing provision and sanitary arrangements. The three central wards were the worst affected with an average of 227 deaths of infants under one year per thousand births, compared with 161 in the outer districts. 44 per cent of these deaths were the result of gastro-intestinal infections and, of these, 8.5 per cent were caused by the zymotic diseases: measles, whooping cough and tuberculosis. Diphtheria also falls into the zymotic category but was not at this time a major problem.[21]

The 1904 outbreak appears to have begun quietly, with thirty-seven cases and five deaths recorded in January. The figures increased steadily month by month, with a few exceptions, and peaked in October when there were 112 cases recorded and seventeen deaths. The August figures are particularly interesting as there were only forty-one cases but the highest number of deaths, nineteen, giving a percentage of deaths to cases rate of 46 per cent. The average fatality rate for the year was 18.1 per cent. The MOH was eager to point out that, although there had been 832 cases and 151 deaths, the death rate (deaths to cases) was less than in the four previous years.[22] (see table 8:1). The following year saw a steady decline in the number of cases although over 470 were recorded. The death total was eighty.

Table 8:1 Diphtheria Mortality in Bradford: 1900-04

Year	Cases	Deaths
1900	109	30
1901	122	28
1902	271	76
1903	196	52
1904	832	151

Table 8:2 Cases and deaths per month: 1904

Month	Cases	Deaths	Month	Cases	Deaths
January	37	5	July	73	10
February	77	12	August	41	19
March	69	10	September	71	14
April	59	7	October	112	17
May	68	13	November	82	15
June	71	12	December	72	17
Totals				832	151

Forty of the recorded deaths occurred in the West Bowling Ward with seventeen in Great Horton and seventeen in neighbouring Little Horton. There were twelve deaths in both the Manningham and East Wards and eleven in East Bowling. The rest of the deaths, that occurred to some degree in all wards, with the exception of North Bierley (West) and Thornton, were fairly evenly spread.[23]

Table 8:3 below gives a clear indication of just how vulnerable the very young were to a fatal attack, with over one third of those aged three years or under dying after contracting the disease. It was also those of school age who were at risk of developing the disease and Dr. Evans quickly noticed this connection. By the end of January he had spotted that sixteen of the twenty-five cases occurred in children attending St Stephen's School in West Bowling and it is here that we now focus our attention.(See figure 8:3) It did, it is true, also attack a number of adjacent schools including Cross Lane Municipal School, St Joseph's, and the municipal schools at Woodroyd and Ryan Street.[24]

Table 8:3 The ages of the victims.

	Attacks	Deaths
Under 3 years of age	96	36
3 years and under 13	622	111
13 years and under 20	51	2
20 years and upwards	63	2
Totals	832	151

The MOH indicated that the 'heavy evidence' that related to the three to thirteen age group suggested that 'the school influence has probably played an important part in the spread of the disease'.[25]

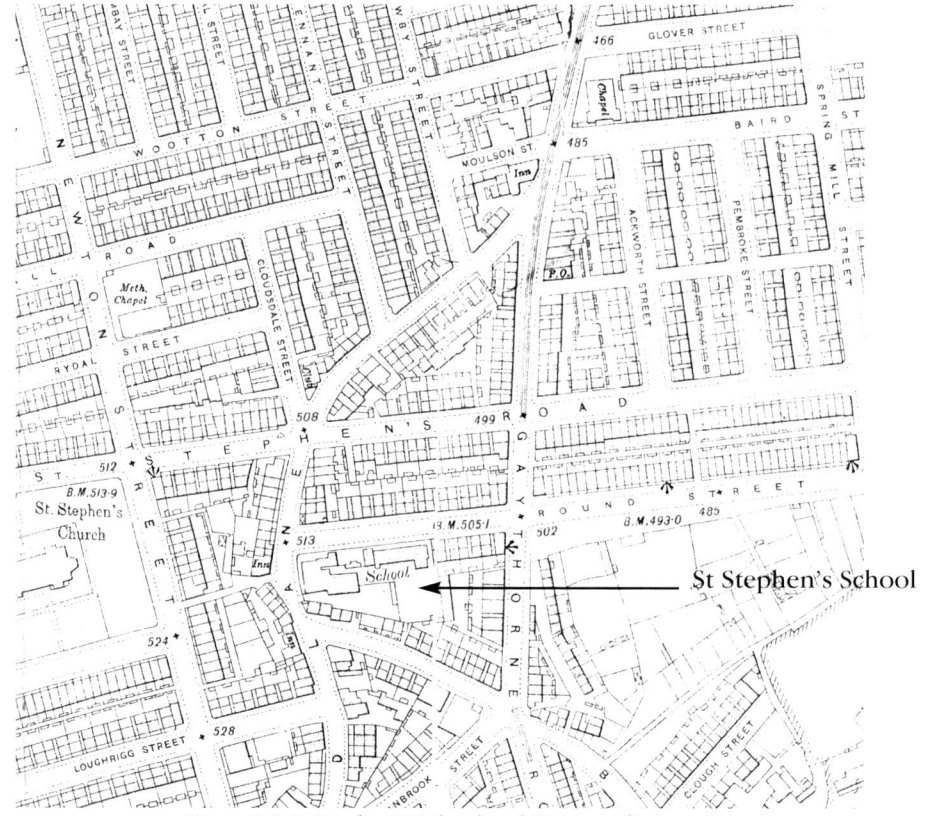

Figure 8:3 St Stephen's School and its immediate environs.
(Ordnance Survey 1908. Surveyed 1889-90. Revised 1905. Sheets CCXXVI.8 & CCXVI 12 . Original scale 1:2500)

West Bowling, where the outbreak was the most severe, is an area that developed from the beginning of the late eighteenth and early nineteenth centuries following the establishment there of Ripley's Dye works and innumerable mills involved in various processes of the textile trade. There was, additionally, Woodroyd Brick Works off Parkside Road, Bowling Parks Brick Works off Birch Lane, and a soap works off Manchester Road. Employment to the east was available for West Bowling residents at the Bowling Ironworks although in general work would be found closer to home.[26] This is apparent when census returns are studied, with evidence, amongst other similar occupations, of wool comb minders, slubbing yarn dyers, stuff warehousemen, dyers labourers, worsted spinners, cashmere weavers, spinning overlookers, cotton dyers and linen finishers.[27]

William Cudworth, in his seminal work on the area, indicated in 1891 that Bowling had been 'much indebted for the employment of many of its inhabitants' to the establishment of the dyeworks. It was in 1812 that George Ripley and his son Edward entered into partnership with William Walton to develop the small business that Walton had begun in 1804. Later generations, especially Sir Henry, Edward's son, continued the business and developed, Ripleyville with 200 workers' houses, 'large and commodious schools,' two phases of almshouses – the later set are still extant, the site for St Bartholmew's Church, and a convalescent home in Rawdon.[28] The iron works were established twenty-four years earlier, in 1788, by John Sturges and Richard Paley. This was a vast undertaking that expanded during the nineteenth-century with tramways bringing coal and ore from, for example, Bierley and Tong. Production ceased in 1898.

Schools Seen as Breeding Grounds

Records and reports relating to the epidemic are disappointingly sparse but the school log books do give us a clue to what life must have been like in the West Bowling area over a hundred years ago. The following are some further entries with, it will be noted, one fatality recorded:

St Stephen's Mixed School West Bowling

29 April: 1904: Seven new cases of diphtheria have been reported this week.
6 May: Five new cases have been reported this week.
11 May: School closed today until 27 inst by order of the Education Committee.
2 June: HMI report: The overcrowding in the main room in which the classes are taught has seriously taxed the efforts of the teachers. [This is of some significance]
21 September: Two cases of diphtheria have been reported.

St Stephen's Infants' School.

29 January 1904: School closed owing to diphtheria.
13 February: Re-opened. Attendance very thin.
29 March. Two cases of epidemic notified. Total of 17.
18 April: Dr. Crowley visited enquiring into the epidemic.
27 April. Four fresh cases of diphtheria during the week.
5 May. Dr. Crowley again visited the school. He examined and swabbed the throats

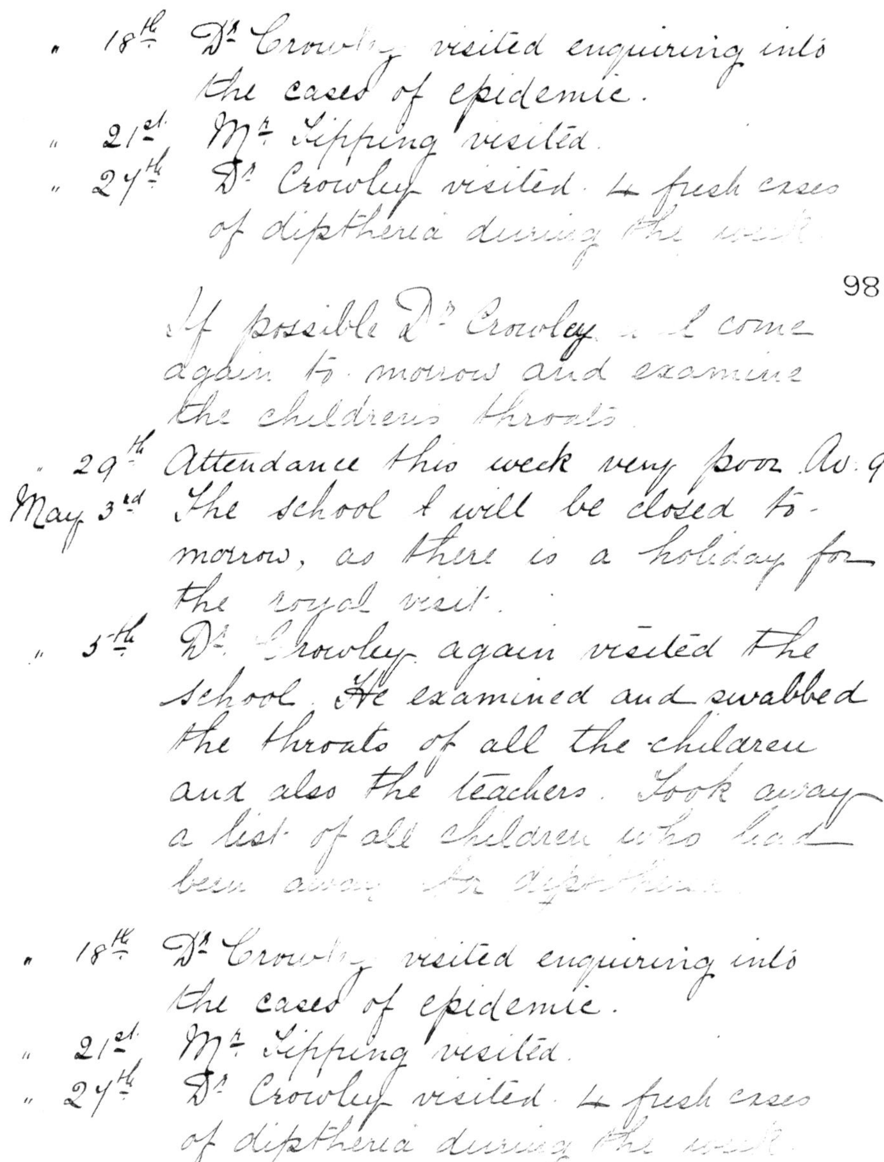

Figure 8:4 Selected log book entries: St Stephen's School. April-May 1904.
(St. Stephen's School, West Bowling)
The Royal visit referred to on 3 May was that of HRH The Princess of Wales.

of all the children and teachers. Took away a list of all the children who had been away with diphtheria.

11 May: Received notice to close the school owing to the prevalence of diphtheria.
17 June: One case of diphtheria reported.
21 June: Dorothy Handel (the child who was reported last week) died.

15 July: The attendance still continues to be poor, and the children who are present are heavy and far from well. [This, I think, can also been seen as a general comment on the health of the children in the area generally, irrespective of diphtheria.]

The penultimate entry recorded above was not the last to report the progress of the epidemic. It is, however, the most poignant. Surprisingly, though, it is the only one to record the death of a pupil and as the school admission registers have not been kept we have no way of knowing of any other deaths amongst the pupils. It has, however, been possible to trace Dorothy via the 1901 census. She was at that time living, aged seven months, with her widowed mother, a shopkeeper, and her elder sister Clara, in Manningham. The family income was supplemented by two married couples who were boarders. Dorothy must have been just under four years old when she died, if the recorded ages are correct. This does seem young to be at school but as she is the only Dorothy Handel in the whole of Bradford we must assume that she and her family moved to West Bowling, where she died. Dorothy was not alone, as the figures already shown indicate, in succumbing to the epidemic. We also know that many other victims were of school age. Schools were in fact, as we have noted, seen as breeding grounds for the disease and were often blamed for its spread. Ventilation was an issue in the St. Stephen's School case and the MOH was of the opinion that:

Defective ventilation of the buildings and the situation of the school itself is to some extent responsible for the spread of the disease amongst its pupils.[29]

Dr. Evans had an interview with the managers and they indicated to him that they were anxious to make some improvements. He also made some suggestions and these included the idea that if the cottages in close proximity to the school were demolished, the external ventilation would be improved. Dr. Evans was in fact clear that although he indicated that the causes of the outbreak were complex, school influence was the chief culprit. He had done a great deal of his research into housing conditions and sanitation, as we shall see, but he was clearly of the opinion that school attendance was the key factor. He did all in his power to see that pupils did not attend school when, for example, siblings were suffering from the disease and circulated a letter to all schools where pupils were affected.[30] He would already be aware of the work that had been done in this field, and would draw strength from it. As Greenwood indicated some thirty years later there is seldom anything dramatic about the business. He believed that there were no great turns of fortune as in, for instance, a water-borne typhoid outbreak.

Greenwood does, however, quote Sir William Power's research in Purbright in Surrey in 1883, which Evans may have known about. Power, a former medical officer to the Local Government Board, found that, relative to other age groups, those of school age were the most likely to be the first to be attacked in the household. They were attacked at twice the rate of children who were no longer attending school. When cases had already occurred in the family, the incidence of attack upon the older children was not much lower than upon those of school age. He noted that 'the data were few' but sufficient, and urged that 'the indication

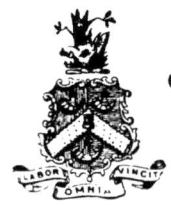

OFFICER OF HEALTH'S DEPARTMENT.

TOWN HALL,

BRADFORD, 190

Dear Sir,

I beg to inform you that there is a case of dangerous Infectious Disease at the house of a pupil attending your School as below.

The child should not be allowed to return to School until you have proper certification that it can do so without danger to itself or to its companions. I would also impress on you that no other child from the infected house should be allowed to attend School until all danger of the disease being spread by it among your pupils has ceased.

I am, yours truly,

W. ARNOLD EVANS,

Medical Officer of Health.

NAME. ADDRESS.

N.B.—In addition to those infectious diseases which are notified to the Sanitary Authority, and about which I am enabled to give you information as above, there are others of a no less infectious character which are not notified. Among these are Measles and Whooping Cough, which are at times widely prevalent, and cause a good many deaths. The same care should be exercised with regard to children and premises infected by these diseases, as is called for in the case of the diseases to which my letter above refers. Your careful supervision to prevent these diseases among your pupils will be of the greatest service.

Figure 8:5 The Medical Officer of Health's letter to headteachers, 1904
(West Yorkshire Archive Service: Bradford. Ref: BB2/2/11)

which they furnish is too uniform to be mistaken'.[31] There were others, such as Shirley Murphy, whom Hardy quotes as showing that notifications for diphtheria (and scarlet fever) declined in London during the August school holiday period.[32] However, further research by E. W. Goodhall found no evidence to show a relationship between school-closure and the incidence of either scarlet fever or diphtheria.[33] It could, I suppose, be argued that the pupils would still be in contact with each other even if the school were closed, although they may be playing in the open air.

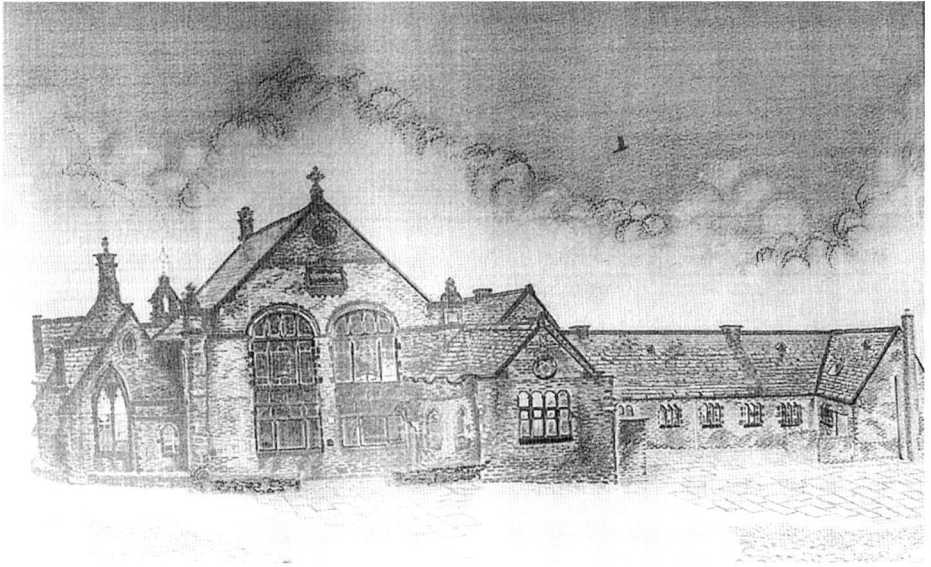

Figure 8:6 St. Stephen's School: The original building
(Courtesy St. Stephen's Primary School)

This undated illustration shows the 1870 building of Bowling Church School, designed by Thomas Healey. It was replaced in 1985 by the current premises in Gaythorne Road.

What then of the MOH's research into the housing and sanitation provision? The area of West Bowling where the worst of the outbreak occurred was developed greatly in the late nineteenth century and many of those living in the area worked at the nearby Bowling Iron works, brickworks or dye works. Most of the houses were of the through variety, though clearly not all, with a yard and an outside privy or WC. It is not clear from the MOH's report just how many of the houses had ashpits or privy middens but he does indicate that it would be advisable to have them emptied 'more frequently that at present'.[34] He is clear, though, that any faults in house construction, or faulty conditions of the privies, were not the cause of the outbreak. In fact in the 832 premises where diphtheria cases occurred - a figure that gives us some idea of the spread of the disease, 696 had satisfactory sanitary conditions. The rest had defects with sink waste pipes, drainage and fall pipes. In ten houses only were the privy and ashpit in a 'foul condition' and only three houses discovered to be in a 'filthy condition'. Two were overcrowded. This is clearly not a desperate picture, especially when compared with conditions

Cruel Lives

discussed in previous chapters.

There was, as indicated in table 8:2 (p.115), a decline in the number of cases by the end of the year from a peak in October. The new-year, 1905, did not, however, see an end of the cases and by December 1905 a further 460 or so cases had been notified, and this figure includes around eighty deaths. A figure that must have continued to give concern, especially as, for example, each year between 1893 and 1901 saw no more than around thirty-five diphtheria deaths. The problem was still, perhaps, that people did not seek medical help soon enough. Bradford was not alone in this respect for as late as 1918, in Leeds, William Angus, the MOH, was complaining that:

There is still a regrettably high number of deaths mostly due to delay in applying energetic treatment…In the successful treatment of diphtheria every day counts.[35]

Chapter Nine

An Unwelcome Present from Scarborough
The 1932 Denby Dale Typhoid Outbreak

The people of Denby Dale and Cumberworth had been drinking contaminated water for many years prior to the outbreak that was to have such a devastating effect on the area, and their lives, in the autumn of 1932. However, it wasn't until typhoid fever arrived in the district that anyone was aware of the fact that waste from a primitive sewerage system had been entering a spring supplying water to the Square Wood reservoir.

The story begins when a twenty-one year old woman, a resident of Quaker Bottom, a small community centred around the Friends' Meeting House at High Flatts to the west of Denby Dale, returned from a holiday in Scarborough in late August. She was unknowingly a typhoid carrier, and it was 17 September before her case was notified.[1] Suddenly the system that had hidden its deadly secret for so many years was finally exposed. This, then, was the beginning of the Denby, Cumberworth and district typhoid outbreak that was to infect seventy-five people in the area and claim twelve of their lives.

Typhoid, often referred to as enteric fever, is a bacterial disease that is spread, like cholera, by water fouled by the faeces of typhoid sufferers or carriers, contaminated food, unwashed hands and occasionally milk.[2] In concise terms, then, the bacteria is spread, as Gill and others indicate, "faeco-orally".[3] It is a disease associated with dirt rather than poverty. The causative organism is *salmonella typhi* harboured in human faeces. The bacillus multiplies in the blood stream and causes a high continuous fever, often accompanied by a rash, and profuse diarrhoea.[4] It can be carried from person to person, perhaps by a person preparing food, who could themselves often be immune. The microbe, after an individual's recovery, can hide in the gall bladder from where it has access to the gut and is excreted in faeces.[5] Healthy people could, therefore, be carriers. This, indicates Wohl, 'added to the mystery of the disease'.[6]

Perhaps the most notorious case concerning a lethal carrier is that of Mary Mallon, born in 1869, an Irish immigrant to the United States of America who infected around forty people, three of whom died. Mallon, who became well known under her nickname of 'Typhoid Mary' had, it was found, an employment history that showed that typhoid had followed her from job to job. After three years in hospital she was released on the understanding that she did not work in the preparation

Cruel Lives

of food. However, she returned to cooking under an assumed name (Mrs. Brown) in 1915 and infected twenty-five people in a maternity hospital. She was arrested and retained in a hospital until her death in 1938.[7]

The disease unlike typhus with which, as we have heard, it was often confused and not recorded separately from until 1869, continued as a major scourge throughout the nineteenth century. However, again unlike typhus, it affected all classes. Typhus, spread by faeces of the body louse, found a home chiefly in overcrowded slum areas where poverty was commonplace. Typhoid, as history often reminds us, entered the homes of rich and poor alike. Prince Albert, it is generally agreed, died of it in 1861 and the Prince of Wales, the future Edward Vll nearly died of it ten years later after staying with the Earl of Londesborough in the North Riding. The prince's groom and the Earl of Chesterfield, who had also been a guest, died from the disease.[8] The provision of sewers that helped to reduce the number of typhus deaths, may, argues Wohl, have actually increased the number of typhoid deaths. Early sewers usually discharged their infected filth into rivers that were often a major source of drinking water.[9]

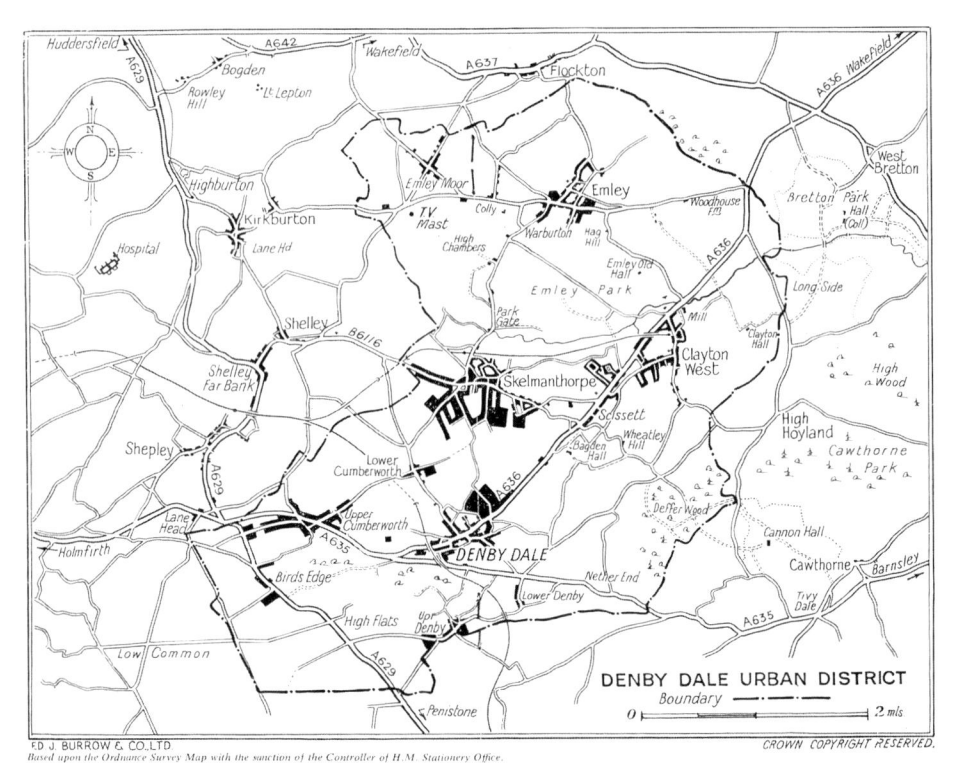

Figure 9:1 Denby Dale and the surrounding villages.
(Denby Dale Urban District Council Guide book. 1972)

Denby Dale is shown here at the heart of the urban district that was formed out of four smaller authorities in 1937. The Denby Dale Urban District then became part of Kirklees Council in 1974. It was in the former Denby and Cumberworth Council area that the typhoid outbreak held its grip.

As in the case of cholera there was, initially, some difference of opinion amongst the medical profession as to exactly how typhoid was carried. Long before the research of William Budd, begun in 1839, into the aetiology of typhoid, the link between typhoid and bad drainage was seen along miasmic principles.[10] His first investigation centred around a well in Clifton, Bristol. He noted that an outbreak occurred in thirteen houses all drawing water from the same well; in his second investigation in Cowbridge, Somerset, again a well was suspected. Here visitors to a ball had stayed at a hotel, where two days earlier a man recovering from typhoid had stayed. The water was drawn near to where the hotel drains were located.

The third case finally convinced him that sewage-tainted water was the cause of many outbreaks of the disease. A fellow doctor, Henry Grace, the father of the famous cricketer, drew his attention to an outbreak in some farm cottages near Bristol. The disease had its origins with a man who had worked in the sewers and lived in a house that had drains that emptied directly into a stream. The results were at last accepted, and by 1860 wells suspected of being polluted were systematically sealed.[11]

The death rate began to fall but it was not until improvements in the water supply and the development of a vaccine against typhoid was developed in 1898 that typhoid outbreaks, and the death rate from the disease, fell even more significantly. The death rate from the disease in England and Wales in the decade 1891-1900 was virtually half that of 1871-80. When using precise years as an example the figures appear even more dramatic. We find that in 1860, the number of deaths attributable to typhoid was 9,185 but by 1910 the figure was down to 1,889.[12] It is, therefore, even more surprising that Denby Dale and its surrounding area should be so badly affected by what was predominately a disease that belonged to the previous century.

The First Signs

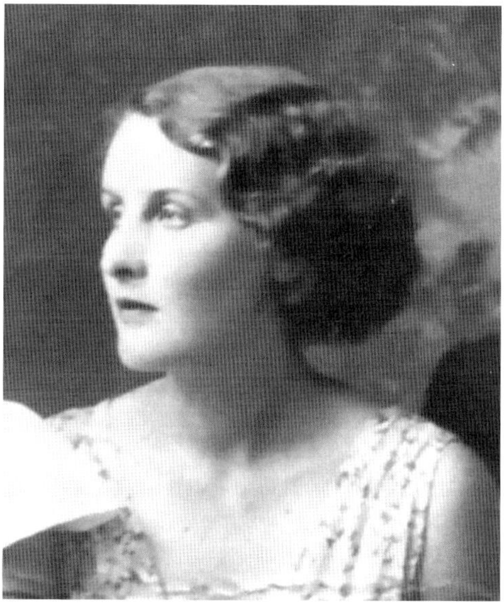

Our story unfolds in the late summer of 1932. People from Denby Dale and Cumberworth, along with those from the surrounding areas had by now returned from their summer holidays and the mills were operational again. Scarborough was a favourite resort for many from the area, who also enjoyed day trips there by train or coach. It was known as a spa town and many enjoyed 'taking the water' whilst on holiday. One of those who spent some time in the Scarborough area during that year was Kate, known as Kitty, Robson who lived in Quaker Bottom at

Figure 9:2 Kitty Robson aged around twenty-one. *(Courtesy of James Anderson)*

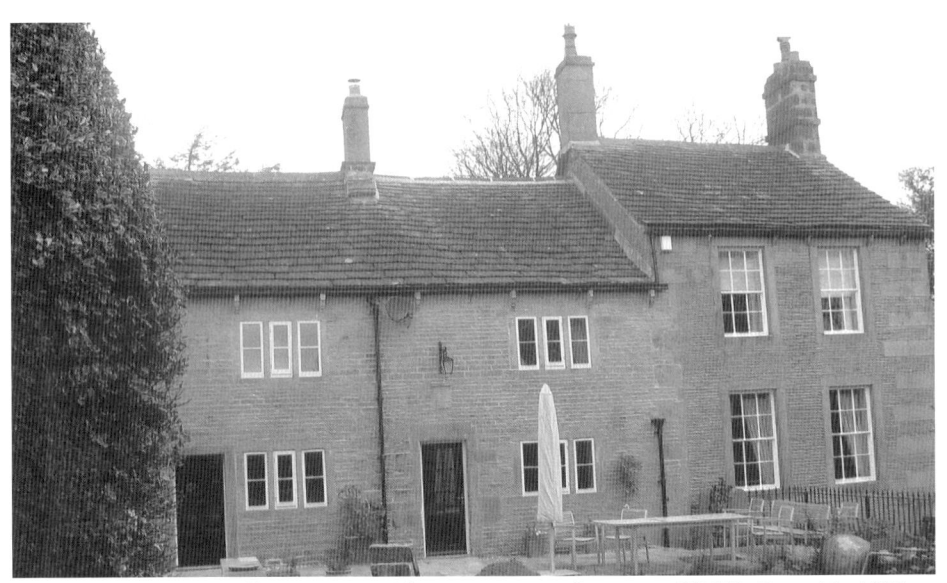

Figure 9:3 'Green Hollows' in 2011. The property was known as 'Middle House' in 1932
(With the permission of William and Susan Cooper)

'Middle House', a property known as 'Green Hollows' since the 1980s.[13] Kate's name was not publicised at the time of the outbreak but it is now known that she was the young woman in question.[14] She is the central, though totally innocent, figure in our story.

Kate Elizabeth Robson was born in Hull on 27 July 1911, the daughter of William Tuke Robson and his wife Grace Beatrice (née Brittain). Her father, who was born in Huddersfield, was at the time of Kitty's birth working as a tramways engineer for Hull Corporation. When the family returned to Huddersfield after William became manager of Huddersfield Corporation public transport, they settled in High Flatts where the family home was next door to the Quaker Meeting House. They do not appear, however, to have been members of the Society of Friends despite Kitty's father having a strong Quaker name, Tuke, as his second forename.[15] In November 1934 Kitty married Richard Harry Tilling, who was born in Surrey in 1904, at Penistone. A daughter, Tessa, was born in 1937. Kitty died at Sutton in Surrey in November 1987.[16]

The meeting house continues today to be a focal point for the community and is an exceptionally attractive building. Meetings appear to have been held, initially in a barn, at what is now known as Quaker Bottom, (a name that appears to have been acquired during the nineteenth century) since around the time of King Charles's execution in 1649. By the end of the century the barn had become established, following alterations, as a permanent Meeting House. More work was done around 1754 that probably involved raising the walls and creating a gallery. Further alterations were carried out on at least four occasions during the nineteenth century. Other buildings within the vicinity of to the Meeting House have included a boarding school established in the 1740s for fifty boys; a day school, a home for 'the restoration of inebriate women of the working and middle

An Unwelcome Present from Scarborough

classes', and a guest house linked to the adult school that met there for courses.[17]

Whether Kitty Robson was infected with the typhoid microbe whilst on holiday, or was already a carrier whose secret was suddenly to be found out, we cannot be sure. The first signs that anything was amiss coincided with the usual incubation period of two weeks, so it is likely that the disease entered Kitty's system at the end of her holiday. She was then ill for a number of days before typhoid was confirmed and notified on 17 September. By that time others had drunk the infected water from Square Wood Reservoir, infected as we learn later by microbes from her faeces, and the Denby and Cumberworth typhoid epidemic was under way. It was soon realised that the drinking water had been infected with human sewage and the supply from Square Wood was immediately cut off. At this stage, though, no one had linked a young woman from Quaker Bottom directly with the outbreak.

A Plague Grips the Village

It was, however, over four weeks later that the first story relating to the 'Terrible Denby Dale Fever Toll' appeared in the local newspapers.[18] Even then, Kitty's part in the story had not come to light. That was a secret waiting to be told. The village, the *Holmfirth and District Express* reported on 22 October, was in the grip of a plague. The fever was raging and the outbreak had already resulted in the deaths of three women, who were all mothers of families living in the village. They were named as Helen Brook, J. Crosland (sic) and R. Laundon.[19] Further research has unearthed more details of names and addresses of these early victims. Annie Crossland of Syke House, who died at Meltham Hospital, was buried at St John's

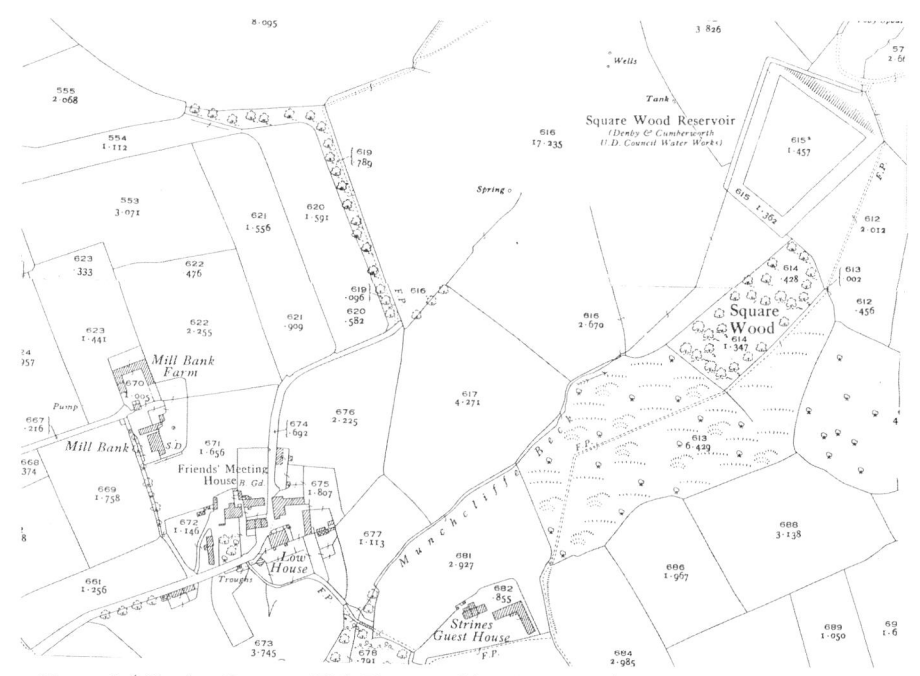

Figure 9:4 Quaker Bottom, High Flatts, and its situation above Square Wood Reservoir.
(Ordnance Survey, 1931 sheets CCLXXIII 2&6. Original scale 1:2500)

Church, Denby, on the 21 October.[20] Helen Brook is, I believe, Ellen Brook of a farm at Leak Hall, as her death is recorded in the Cumberworth Church burial register on the day of her funeral, 22 October. Amy Laundon, who died at Mill Hill Fever Hospital, was buried on the same day, but in Denby.[21] The initial R in the newspaper reports refers to Mrs. Laundon's husband's name, Redfearn, as shown in the electoral roll.[22]

We have little information in relation to these women but we can assume, I think, that Amy Laundon lived at Co-operative Terrace (now Garden Terrace) as her husband and son were taken from there in November to Meltham Hospital.[23] Thirty-five cases were in hospital and three or four people were hovering between life and death.[24] A week later the death of Lister Stead Peace, aged seventy-two, the president of Denby Dale and District Free Church Council was announced. His niece, Connie Fisher, was ill in Meltham Hospital[25]

The *Huddersfield Weekly Examiner*, published on 22 October, also carried detailed news from Denby Dale but led with a somewhat optimistic sub-heading that informed readers that the 'infection was on the wane.'[26] The MOH for the Denby and Cumberworth Urban District, Dr. J.T. Bleasdell, had reported to the council at a meeting two days earlier that forty-five cases had been admitted to four isolation hospitals. These were at Penistone, Kirkburton, Meltham and Huddersfield. Taxis were provided, courtesy of the council, for family members visiting the hospitals, by the local firm of Fred and Edwin Hirst of Denby Dale.[27] The local papers also carried details of the patients in each of the four hospitals. These were updated on a daily basis and often this was the only way that friends and relatives could hear what progress, or otherwise, the patients were making. Often messages for relatives were also published in the papers. On 19 November, for example, the *Huddersfield Examiner* reported from Penistone Hospital that:

The matron of this hospital announces that the following require outdoor clothing: Harold Brown, Henry Stephenson, Nancy Hartley and Agnes Kitson.

Earlier in the month, on the first Thursday, the paper had published the following lists, chosen here as a random example, from the four hospitals.

Table 9:1 Denby Dale typhoid outbreak hospital lists: 3 November 1932[28]

Mill Hill Hospital

Frank Hobson, 1 Sunnybank, Denby Dale, *seriously ill.*
Mildred Stanger, High Street, D D, *seriously ill.*
Vincent Bedford, Wakefield Road, D D, *progressing favourably.*
Cyril Lockwood, 3 Dean View, D D, *progressing favourably.*
Frank Holmes, Wall Royds, Kaye Lane, D D, *progressing favourably.*
Dorothy Littlewood, 1 Victoria Terrace, D D, *seriously ill*
Margaret Shepley, School House, D D, *seriously ill.*
Lena and Eva Horn, Wood Nook, D D, *progressing favourably.*
Joseph Briggs, High Street, D D, *seriously ill.*

Frank Winston Peace, Brentwood, Upper Cumberworth, *progressing favourably.*
Gertrude Ellis, Ing Cottage, Wakefield Road, Denby Dale, *progressing favourably.*
Mabel Howard, Field House, D D, *progressing favourably.*
Roy Crossland, North View, D D, *seriously ill.*
Mona Stevenson, Leak Hall Farm, D D, *seriously ill.*
Ida Walker, Hartley View, D D, *progressing favourably.*
Joyce Crossland, North View, D D, *progressing favourably.*
Gertrude Lockwood, High street, D D, *progressing favourably.*
Mary Parker, Park View, D D, *progressing favourably.*
Edith Stevenson, High Street, D D, *seriously ill.*

Meltham Isolation Hospital

Norman Hirst, Clayton West, *very serious.*
Alice Stanger, High Street, Denby Dale, *very serious.*
Connie Fisher, Exley Gate, D D, *slight improvement.*
Elizabeth George, Close Lane, D D, *slight improvement.*
Bessie Kitson, West Leigh, D D, *making satisfactory progress.*
Betty Morris, Norman Croft, D D, *slight improvement.*
Mrs Ibbotson, Park Mill, Clayton West, *not as well.*
Kathleen Ibbotson (a baby) Park Mill, Clayton West, *making satisfactory progress.*
George T Firth, Victoria Terrace, D D, *slight improvement.*
Fred Wainwright, High Street, D D, *very serious.**
Frank Priest, D D, *very serious.*
Edna Tingle, Penistone, *very serious.**
Mabel Lockwood, Wakefield Road, D D, *making satisfactory progress.*
Phyllis Stringer, Kingussie House, D D, *comfortable.*
George A Wood, D D, *slight improvement.*
Mabel Peace, D D, *comfortable.*
James W Lockwood, School Terrace, D D, *making satisfactory progress.*

Penistone Isolation Hospital

Harold Brown, Polygon Terrace, Denby Dale, *satisfactory.*
Jack Turton, Norman Road, D D, *dangerous, parents may visit.*
Agnes Kitson, West Leigh, *satisfactory.*
Nancy Hartley, Morley Bottom, D D, *progressing favourably.*
Henry Stephenson, High Street, *satisfactory.*
Keith Lockwood (a baby) Wakefield Road, D D, *satisfactory.*
Nurse Johnson (a member of the hospital staff who became infected in the course of her work) *satisfactory.*

Kirkburton

Mrs Andrews, High Street, Denby Dale, *comfortable.*
Leslie Priest, School Terrace, D D, *comfortable.*
Frank and Mrs Totten, Smithroyd, D D, *satisfactory,*
Edna Sharp Halls, Hartcliffe View, D D, *slight improvement*
William Peace, North View, Upper Cumberworth, *slight improvement, good night.*

Kathleen Hanson, Wesley Terrace, D D, *improvement.*
Edith Firth, Exley Gate, D D, *satisfactory.*
Arthy Beevers, Smithroyd, D D, *slight improvement, good night.**
Frank Wood, West End, Skelmanthorpe, *very ill but slight improvement.*
Ronald Fisher, Lodge Street, Skelmanthorpe, *very ill but slight improvement.*
Jack Bilcliffe, Elm Street, Skelmanthorpe, *very ill but slight improvement.*

* Later added to the listed of fatalities[29]

The MOH also gave a description of a sample of water tested by the county bacteriologist that showed that the water from Square Wood was polluted.[30] Council members were also informed at the meeting by Dr. Bleasdell that the disease was on the wane and that with the support of the County Council every effort was being made to correct the source of the trouble. The press and public were excluded from this meeting, by the chairman of the council, John Hinchliffe. There was a good deal of anger at this decision, as can be imagined, and comments such as 'we have every right, as rate-payers,to be informed officially of the true state of affairs'.[31] Even the headteacher of the Denby Dale District Council School, Sam Shepley, who was also a councillor, was drawn into expressing an opinion, perhaps unwisely, when reporters from the *Barnsley Chronicle* visited the school. He was quoted as saying that:

The majority of people in the village are rather indignant over the fact that the council have not been a little more open in their communications with them[32]

Shepley was clearly, however, speaking from the heart. One of the patients listed in the *Huddersfield Examiner*, a few days earlier on 22 October, as suffering from the disease in Mill Hill Hospital, Huddersfield was his daughter Margaret of School House, Denby Dale. She was said to be progressing satisfactorily but was still listed with others at Mill Hill, in the paper four weeks later.[33]

The council was also been criticised in the daily edition of the *Huddersfield Examiner* on 19 and 20 October. The Clerk to the Council, G.S.Mosley, writing on behalf of the council, was clearly annoyed by the 'preposterous reports' relating to the outbreak that had appeared in the paper. Things were bad enough, he believed, without such reporting and they were 'gravely concerned' by what they read. During his ten years as clerk there had not been a healthier district in England. Sixty per cent, or around five hundred, of the houses were now on the water carriage system. It is, however, appropriate to add here that as in other villages and towns, there were still many (541) earth closets in the district. The editor was quick to add a footnote to the clerk's letter, claiming that he was at a loss to discover what these preposterous reports were! [34]

When the water from Square Wood was cut off, the community received its supplies from other local reservoirs. At the council offices of the Denby and Cumberworth Urban District Council, that served a population of 3,396 (1931 census), it was stated that the infected reservoir was being cleared and cleaned.[36]

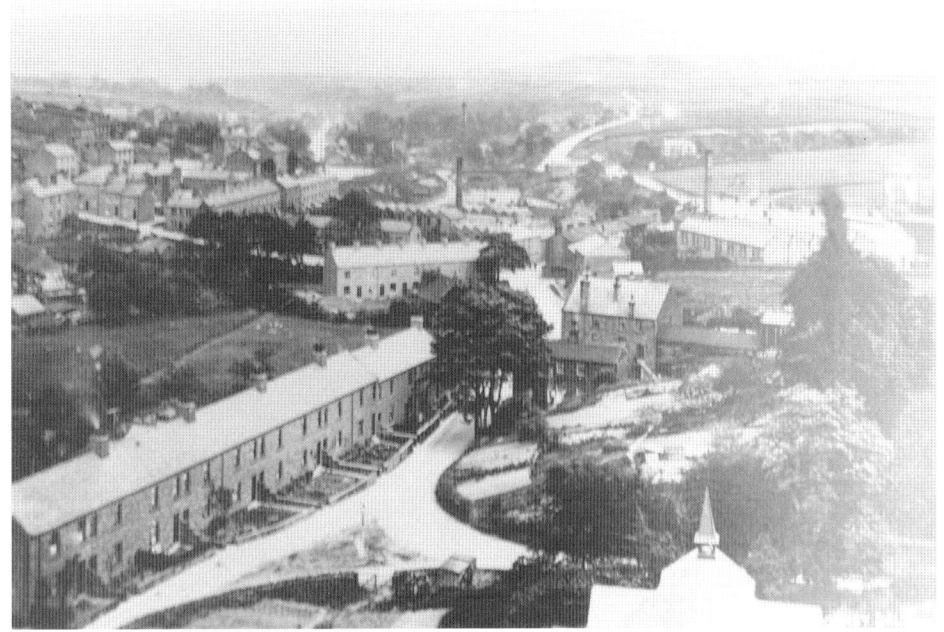

Figure 9:5 Denby Dale from the west c1922.
(Stanley Sheead collection)

Dearnside and Springfield Mills are shown in the centre of the picture. The cupola of the former wood and corrugated iron Holy Trinity Church, consecrated in 1893, can be seen in the foreground. The original building was replaced in 1939 by the building in use today.[35]

It was also reported, somewhat precipitately, that 'it is expected that within a week it will be safe to supply from it'.[37] Many, however, preferred to take water from private sources such as Kenyon's Mill, and the local gas works. There is, however, an interesting side story related to woollen manufacturers, Kenyon's, who along with Hinchliffe's at Hartcliffe Mills, and Brownhills were major employers in the community and had all been established during the period 1850-68.[38] An employee of the firm was ill with typhoid in a Glasgow hospital and it is difficult to imagine that those using the mill's water supply were aware of this fact.[39]

Locals also supplemented their liquid intake with whisky, as an apparent protection against the typhoid. It was reported that so great had been the demand for the spirit in local public-houses that the publicans had to telephone for extra supplies![40] In fact, when a reporter and a colleague from the *Barnsley Chronicle* visited the area around 25 October and turned to 'that infallible source of gossip', the village pub, they found many to be deserted. At the White Hart Hotel they were, however, told by a lady that whisky sales had soared and that 'I never thought that people could drink so much of it'.[41] At the Prospect Hotel A.H. Addy, the licensee, reported on 19 October that his shelves were cleared of whisky.[42]

Other trade quickly began to suffer, as people were frightened to venture into the local shops and avoided contact with neighbours and friends. This was despite the fact that people were reassured that there was no danger of 'picking up' typhoid when walking about. This wasn't quite the 'economic disaster' that was to befall

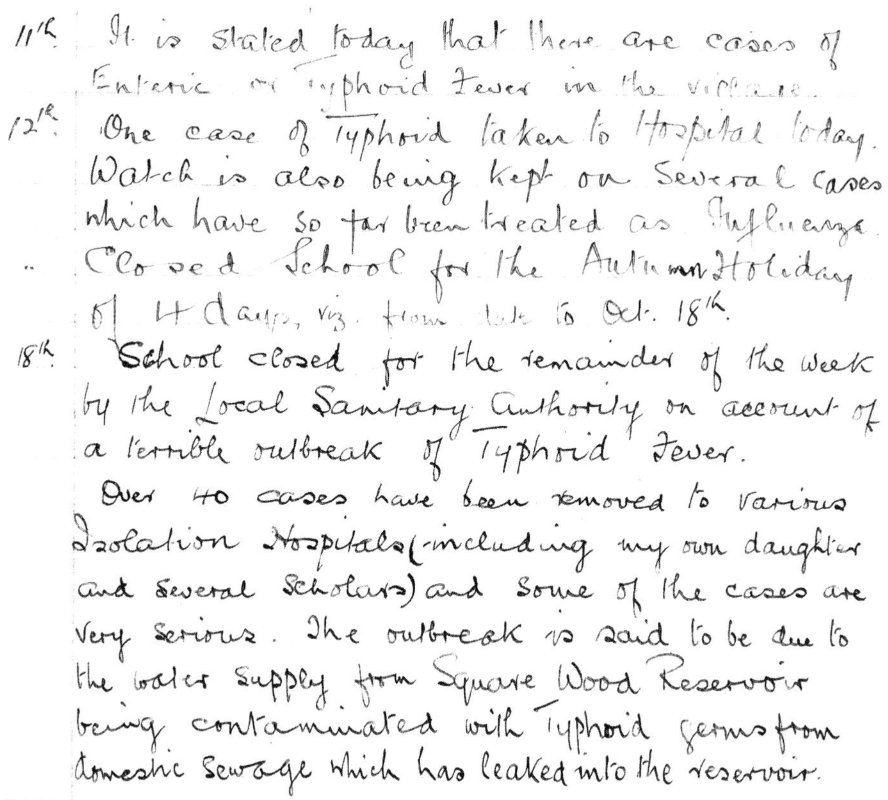

> 11th. It is stated today that there are cases of Enteric or Typhoid Fever in the village.
>
> 12th. One case of Typhoid taken to Hospital today. Watch is also being kept on several cases which have so far been treated as Influenza. Closed School for the Autumn Holiday of 4 days, viz. from ... to Oct. 18th.
>
> 18th. School closed for the remainder of the week by the Local Sanitary Authority on account of a terrible outbreak of Typhoid Fever. Over 40 cases have been removed to various Isolation Hospitals (including my own daughter and several Scholars) and some of the cases are very serious. The outbreak is said to be due to the water supply from Square Wood Reservoir being contaminated with Typhoid germs from domestic sewage which has leaked into the reservoir.

Figure 9:6 The Denby Dale School log book. October 1932
(West Yorkshire Archive Service, Kirklees. Ref: CW/E/DD/6)

Malton when typhoid struck there during late October but many shopkeepers and farmers were suffering.[43] Local farmers, especially, were finding it difficult to sell their milk as people feared infection from the cows that had been grazing in the fields surrounding the polluted reservoir.[44] Milk, and even butter, was being boiled.[45] Not surprisingly it was reported that some of the local people and the shopkeepers were showing signs of 'frayed nerves'. A further precaution was taken as early as 18 September when the school closed. Sam Shepley, the headteacher of the elementary school (for pupils aged seven to fourteen) recorded in the log book on 18 October that:

School closed for the remainder of the week by the local sanitary authority, on account of a terrible outbreak of typhoid fever.

He had already recorded, on 11 October, and on the following day, that 'watch is being kept on several cases' of typhoid in the village. He reported that some of his pupils, (eleven by 21 October) including his own daughter, had been removed to the isolation hospitals. He added that some of the cases were very serious.

The school eventually re-opened on 24 October and this arrangement was not very popular with the local people. It was considered to be an absurd decision by the West Riding County Council Education Committee whilst the epidemic was raging.

Clearly many refused to accept the decision and the attendance was but seventy out of the 246 on the school registers.[46] The protests did, however, have some effect as the school closed again on 31 October for, initially, two weeks. Only eighteen pupils had attended the previous Friday.[47]

A similar situation was reported by the headteacher of the Victoria Hall Council Infants' School, Florence Bransgrove. The closure pattern was identical to the older pupils' school as was the attendance. On 28 October only seven pupils' attended out of a school roll of eighty. Earlier in the week Miss Bransgrove had recorded that there was 'still not a regular supply of water' at the school.

When the schools reopened on 21 November there were still issues to be dealt with beyond the usual day-to-day management of the schools. On the day that the infants' school opened three pupils were sent home because there had been a recent outbreak of the fever in their homes. At the older children's school the head was in the process of writing to each home where parents were still nervous and keeping their children from school to point out that all precautions were being taken. Both headeachers would have other issues to consider during the next few years. The infants' school closed for good on 13 April 1933 and the children and staff, including the headteacher (as a class teacher) transferred to the Denby Dale Council school. They joined Sam Shepley for just a year as he retired on 31 May 1934 after thirty-one years as headteacher of the school.[48] He was succeeded by Francis Taylor from Beaker Hill School in Barnsley.[49]

It is easy to understand the parents' defiance, especially as they would find more bad news falling through their letter boxes or when collecting their paper on 29 October. The *Holmfirth Express* introduced its lengthy article on the outbreak with the heading 'Typhoid Death Drama' and as a sub-heading made it clear that the epidemic was now taking lives. Five local people had died from the epidemic in the space of two weeks. Sixty-two people were in hospital. The latest victim was Thomas Noble, aged sixty-one, of Hartcliffe View, Denby Dale. He was a local councillor and, somewhat ironically, a member of the waterworks committee that controlled the offending reservoir.

The Epidemic's Lethal Journey Continues

The paper continued to report the epidemic in a moderate manner but, not surprisingly, was eager to stress the human side of things. Stories relating to two of the victims prove this point. Thomas Noble's younger son, Robert, lived at Swinton, Manchester and on hearing that his father was dying in Meltham Hospital, made a 'dramatic dash' to the hospital, perhaps by bus and train. He was greeted at the hospital door by a nurse who told him that his father had just died. A further story concerned Mrs. Mary Emma Parker of Park View, Denby Dale (referred to as Barker in the *Holmfirth Express*)[50] who was seriously ill in the Huddersfield Hospital. She was unaware that as she asked visitors if her husband and brother were alright, her brother Ernest Lockwood, thirty-one, also of Park View, was being buried in the graveyard of St Nicholas's Church, Cumberworth.[51] A week later readers were made aware of 'one of the most moving episodes of the typhoid

THE DENBY DALE EPIDEMIC

A PATIENT LOSES HER HUSBAND

THE SIXTH DEATH

WHAT THE VILLAGERS WANT TO KNOW

DEATH has claimed still another victim of the Denby Dale typhoid epidemic. Yesterday afternoon Mr. George Parker (32), of Park View, Denby Dale, passed away in Mill Hill Isolation Hospital, Huddersfield.

This, the sixth death, is the most tragic episode of the village typhoid drama. Mr. Parker's young wife at present lies in the ward next to that in which her husband died. She, too, is a victim of the disease. Her brother, Ernest Lockwood, died from the fever over a week ago.

She has still to be informed that her husband and her brother are dead.

She is stated to have said to friends who have visited her in hospital: "I hope that my husband and my brother are all right."

Two more cases were taken to hospital yesterday. They are Frank Priest, of Denby Dale, and Edna Tingle, of Penistone. It is believed that Edna Tingle contracted the disease in Denby Dale.

To-day both schools in the village were closed. The children have been given a fortnight's holiday.

THE VILLAGE WATER

The people of Denby Dale are still much concerned about many things, but perhaps most of all about their water supply (writes an "Examiner" representative).

Figure 9:7 The Huddersfield Examiner 2 November 1932

drama'. It was reported that Mrs. Parker's husband George had also died, aged thirty-one. She had, at this stage, not been informed of his death, nor that of her brother. The epidemic was continuing on its lethal journey through Denby Dale and Cumberworth.[52] Further afield at Penistone Hospital, the matron, Miss Butler, reported that they had what was believed to be 'the worst case of typhoid ever admitted to an English hospital'.[53]

George Parker's son Philip, until his death in 2011, still lived in the house in Denby Dale where he was brought up. He was four-and-a-half years old when his father and uncle died. His uncle, Ernest Lockwood, lived next door with parents Arthur and Martha Lockwood. Ernest's sister, Mary Emma, had moved next door when she married George. I was able during early 2011 to talk to Mr. Parker and to his wife Marjorie (née Wood), and learn from them the remarkable fact that between them they lost three close relatives in the epidemic, as Doreen Wood, Mrs. Parker's aunty, had also died from typhoid fever. Doreen was the sister of Marjorie's father Charles. (See figure 9:8)

Readers had learned that the seventh death had been recorded on 3 November when Doreen, aged twenty-one, of Co-operative Terrace, died. Doreen's death brought to the end what the paper described as a 'mother's grim ordeal' at the side of her unconscious daughter in Penistone Hospital. Miss Wood was a fine singer, and member of the choir of Miller Hill Methodist Church. Her minister, the Reverend O.A. Ward had twelve of his congregation in hospital.

More news was beginning to emerge around this time in relation to just how the germs had entered the reservoir. A statement by the council with the following information was attached to the council offices door:

An old rubble land drain has been found in the vicinity of the reservoir which has allowed leakage to escape from the beck into the spring supplying the reservoir, and it has been a source of contamination to the water supply to Denby Dale. Every action is being taken to ensure that no leakage of this kind will take place in the future.[54]

An Unwelcome Present from Scarborough

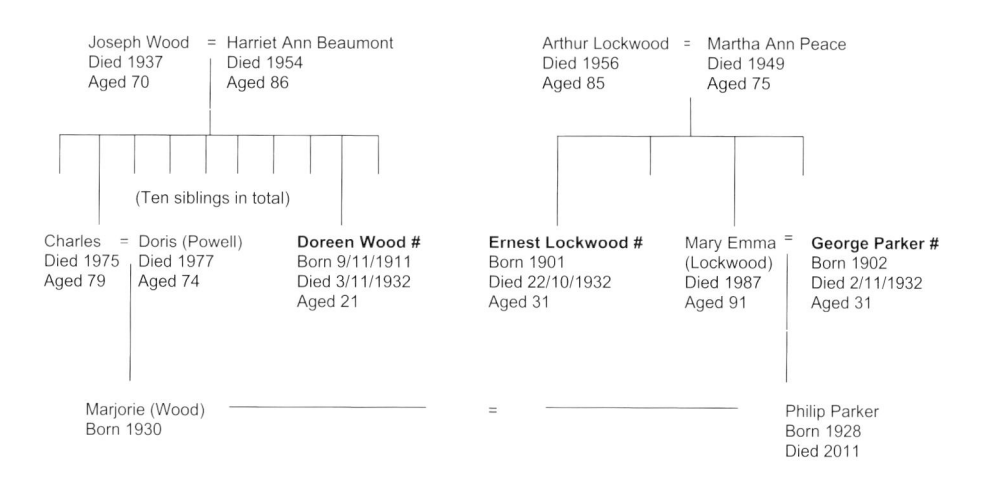

```
Joseph Wood    =  Harriet Ann Beaumont          Arthur Lockwood  =  Martha Ann Peace
Died 1937         Died 1954                      Died 1956            Died 1949
Aged 70           Aged 86                        Aged 85              Aged 75
```

(Ten siblings in total)

Charles = Doris (Powell)	**Doreen Wood #**	**Ernest Lockwood #**	Mary Emma = **George Parker #**
Died 1975 / Died 1977	Born 9/11/1911	Born 1901	(Lockwood) / Born 1902
Aged 79 / Aged 74	Died 3/11/1932	Died 22/10/1932	Died 1987 / Died 2/11/1932
	Aged 21	Aged 31	Aged 91 / Aged 31

Marjorie (Wood) ——————————————— = ——————————————— Philip Parker
Born 1930   Born 1928
                                                                   Died 2011

# denotes the three family members.

Figure 9:8 The Wood, Parker and Lockwood family tree.[55]

This outline family tree shows how the marriage of Philip Parker and Marjorie Wood brought together two families that lost three of their members to typhoid in 1932.

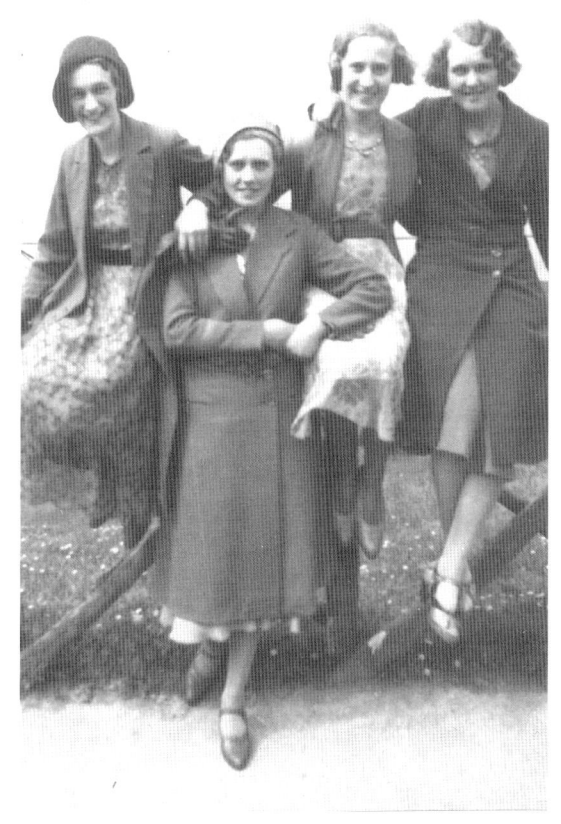

9:9 Doreen Wood c 1929. She is on the far right of the photograph.
(Barry Natton collection)

Doreen's elder sister Marion is second from the left. The others pictured are Doris Crossland (far left) and Phyllis Stringer.

135

The notice was signed by John Hinchliffe J.P. as chairman of the council, the medical officer, and the clerk. It is perhaps worth remembering at this stage just how difficult it must have been for such a small council to deal with such a major issue. It was not until 1938, when Denby Dale Urban District Council was created out of Denby and Cumberworth, Clayton West, Skelmanthorpe and Emley Councils, that officers were able, formally, to work together to gradually improve the area's facilities and share expertise during difficult times.

Residents were also told that the local M.P., C. Glossop, had paid a visit to the area and was perfectly satisfied that the work being done would ensure a satisfactory water supply. The water being drawn from Rusby Wood, that normally fed Cumberworth, was proving to be adequate. Residents were also reassured that there were no immediate plans to re-open Square Wood reservoir. It was, however, agreed later, on 22 December, that the reservoir should be refilled in case of an emergency such as fire.[56] When it was suggested around 29 October by the clerk, G.S. Mosley, that the reservoir could be operational again in two weeks there was a 'storm of protest' from the villagers.

There was also a story with a happy ending reported in the paper that included much praise for Dr. Bleasdell. He had found, late at night, the life of a little girl to be in 'grave danger' when visiting her home. An ambulance was not available so, we read, the doctor wrapped some blankets round her and drove her to Penistone Hospital in his own car. Somewhat paradoxically the same edition of the *Holmfirth Express* carried a sub-heading to the effect that 'the danger was practically at an end'.[57] These were, in fact, the words of the Leeds MOH, Dr. Johnstone Jervis, who wanted to stress that the outbreaks in Denby Dale and Malton (where there had been an even more severe outbreak with 235 cases)[58] had assumed an importance in other districts 'that the position scarcely warrants', as the source of the infection had been traced.[59]

A week later it was reported that the death toll was ten and that sixty-six people were still in hospital. The three most recent deaths were those of Edna Tingle, aged twenty, a Penistone resident who had worked in a Denby Dale mill, Arthy Beevers, 69, a tailor of Smithroyd, Denby Dale, and Fred Wainwright of High Street who was forty-eight. Arthy Beevers, who died in Kirkbuton Hospital, was the organist at Miller Hill Methodist Church, where a new organ had just been installed to commemorate his fifty years' service.[60] He was buried at St. Nicholas's Church on 10 November and is recorded in the register as Arthur, aged sixty-six.[61] Fred Wainwright was a skilled and well-known local billiards player. As well as the suffering directly related to the disease, the outbreak had also caused much poverty in the community. There were no wage earners in some families and people had to put up a 'grim fight' to make ends meet. One man with ten children, two of whom were suffering from typhoid fever, 'scarcely knew where his next meal was coming from.'[62]

One lady with clear memories of the outbreak, Mary Lockwood, is still living in the area. I had the opportunity to meet Mrs. Lockwood (née Priest), who was born in 1912, during the writing of this book. Although aged almost ninety-eight, she was able to recall clearly those desperate weeks almost eighty years ago. She was living with her parents at the time, as were her younger brothers, in School Terrace. Both Mrs. Lockwood's brothers contracted the disease and were confined to the isolation hospitals: Lesley first, to Kirkburton, and then shortly afterwards Frank, to Meltham. The family owned an adjacent fish and chip shop, Priests, that closed during the epidemic 'so we couldn't pass it on'. Mrs. Lockwood, who worked at Z. Hinchliffe's mill in the village as a spinner, recalled that, 'every house down the main road seemed to be affected'.[63]

Startling News

The most startling news, however, had broken in the *Huddersfield Examiner* on 5 November and a week later in the more local paper, the *Holmfirth Express*. Readers were informed that the County MOH, Dr. T.N.V. Potts, had made some remarkable disclosures in the medical journal the *Lancet*. He wrote that:

It does appear that the inhabitants of the village of Denby Dale have been drinking contaminated water for many years.[64]

In his report to the *Lancet*, reported in the papers and in his annual report as County Medical Officer, Dr. Potts was absolutely clear that the infection had its origins at Quaker Bottom, when he wrote in his report that there appeared to be little doubt about the original source of the infection. He confirmed that a woman, aged twenty-one, who had been taking a holiday in or around the seaport town of Scarborough had returned to her home amongst a group of houses situated on the hillside five hundred yards above the Square Wood Reservoir. She was, as we have heard, notified as suffering from typhoid fever on 17 September and from 8 October additional cases began to occur. The Square Wood reservoir had been constructed some forty years earlier and had a capacity of 2,500,000 gallons. It drew its water from springs situated in the gathering ground surrounding the reservoir. These were connected to the reservoir by underground pipelines. It is here that we find the heart of the story.[65]

It appeared, said Dr. Potts, that some years earlier water closets had been installed for the houses at Quaker Bottom and the drainage (the *Huddersfield Examiner* was more to the point and called it sewage!) from these houses was made to discharge into the Munchcliffe Beck (referred to as Dyke in the reports) via the tributary stream. There appears to have been no system of filtering, and waste from the water closets ran untreated into the Munchcliffe Beck via a covered gulley, the tributary stream and, possibly, some underground pipework. The sewage from the houses at Quaker Bottom did not run into a sewerage system, through which waste usually passes to filter beds, but ran into the ground some distance from the houses and the only outlet for it was the beck.[66] Although the evidence is not altogether clear I have, with the help of local farmer David Cook, been able to gain a better understanding of what was a primitive and inadequate system. Whatever sewage disposal method was in place at Quaker Bottom, one thing is clear: infected water found its way into the reservoir via the gulley and the Munchcliffe Beck.

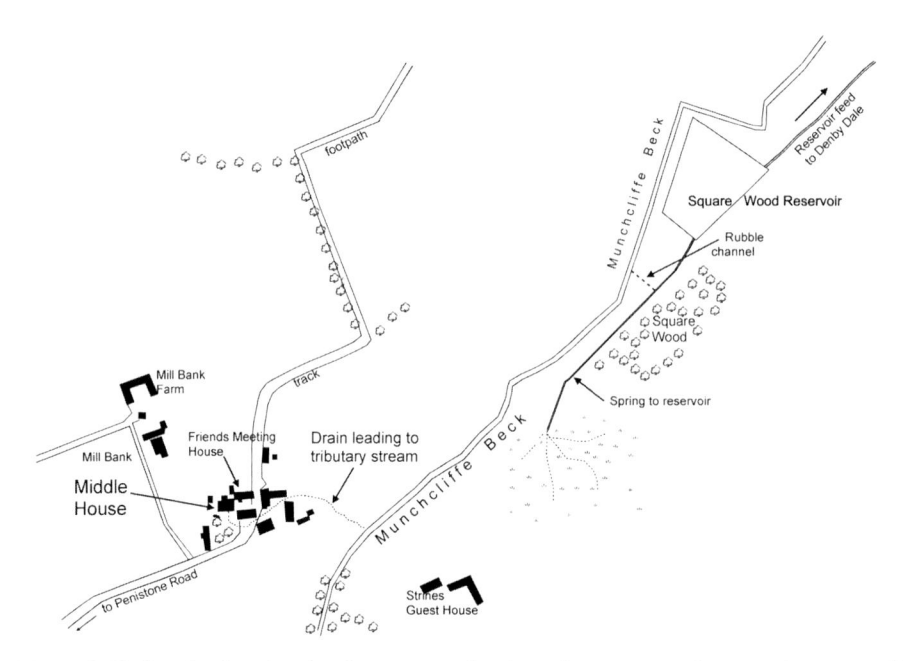

Figure 9:10 Sketch plan showing how contamination of Square Wood Reservoir occurred.[67]
(Based on 1933 mapping and an explanatory sketch by Ron Jackson in 2011)

'Middle House', Kate Robson's home, was renamed 'Green Hollows' in the mid-1980s.[68]

However the system 'worked', we now know that the discharge included germs from the lethal evacuations of the young lady who had enjoyed a holiday in Scarborough. Following Dr. Bleasdell's and a surveyor's visit to the site it was noticed, after careful examination of the sides of the beck, that an old rubble drain was found and this was communicating directly with the main spring supplying the reservoir. The contaminated water was seen to be entering the reservoir's communicating channel. This drain had been installed some time ago to augment, if necessary, the supply of water to the reservoir by using the beck. Helpfully for the council, Dr. Potts was able to add that the existence of this channel between the beck and the nearby spring would not have been known to those who connected the closets to the water carriage system. This news was clearly a shock to the people but what followed was an even greater shock for Dr. Potts had more to say, as had the papers. He indicated that the water had been infected for many years and the eyes of readers would, no doubt, have been quickly drawn to the following paragraph taken from his report and printed in bold type in the *Huddersfield Weekly Examiner:*

It does appear that the inhabitants of Denby Dale village, numbering some 1,400 persons, will have been drinking contaminated water for many years, and had it not been for the advent of the typhoid patient to the house in Quaker Bottom situated above the reservoir, it is likely that this tainted water would have continued to be consumed indefinitely.[69]

Dr. Potts also reiterated in his report the time scale of the microbes' spread. He was clear that the timescale of events was consistent with the suggestion that the young woman from Quaker Bottom was the original source of infection. The danger of further infection was eliminated once the Square Wood supply was cut off, and anti-typhoid vaccine had been supplied. Only by people disregarding 'ordinary preventative' measures was any further risk encountered. When the report was published it was announced that there were still many potential and actual sources of pollution at Square Wood and that the Minister of Health was not prepared to 'concur with the use of this reservoir' until all sources have been investigated. It was, therefore, decided by the council to purchase water from the Dewsbury and Heckmondwike Water Board.[70]

The MOH's report, that covered the year of the outbreak, also contained additional statistics in relation to the urban district. As expected, the typhoid outbreak had pushed the district into equal second place in the county's district councils' death figures. Excluding the county boroughs such as Leeds, Dewsbury, Huddersfield and the like, Denby Dale had a mortality rate of 16.2 per thousand, as had Calverley. Haworth had the highest at 16.7; Greasbrough near Rotherham the lowest at 6.9. In the county's urban districts there had been 16,234 births and 13,687 deaths. In Denby and Cumberworth the balance was reversed with thirty-

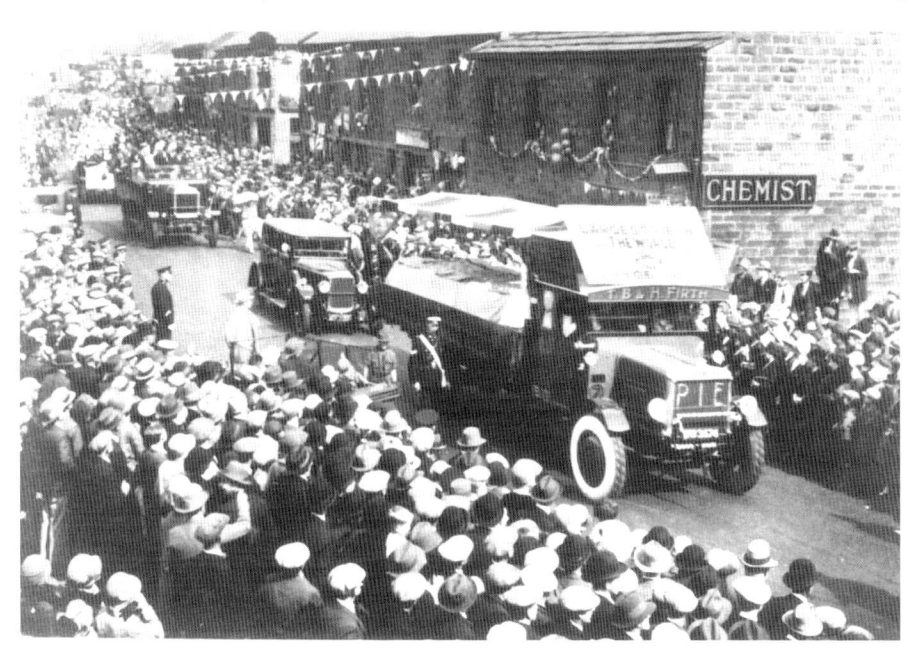

Figure 9:11 Wakefield Road, Denby Dale. Pie Celebrations in 1928.
(Stanley Sheead collection)

A happy occasion, and a well-known part of Denby Dale tradition. The procession was headed by the Denby Dale Prize Band. The headteacher, Sam Shepley, recorded in the school log book that: 'It has been decided to bake the "World's Greatest Pie" in the village. Denby Dale has long been famous for its pies but this one is to eclipse all previous ones in size and weight.'[71] Four years later the town was ravaged by typhoid. Many of those seen here would, no doubt, be infected by the outbreak.

Cruel Lives

seven births and fifty-four deaths. Each year the MOH reports, and certainly those from the nineteenth and early twentieth centuries, tended to include details of some form of epidemic outbreak. This one was no exception with 209 cases of scarlet fever being recorded in Spenborough and, no doubt to the satisfaction of the councillors, only two in Denby and Cumberworth. Scarlet fever, as we have heard elsewhere, was a virulent disease and in the Huddersfield Medical Officer's report for 1933 there is evidence of 547 cases and forty-five deaths from the disease.[72]

This, as we can imagine, was not the end of the story and the council was quickly on the defensive when several untrue and misleading statements were made. A detailed statement was handed to the press following a special meeting, from which reporters were again excluded, on 3 November. The council was eager to point out that the water supplies from Square Wood and Rusby Wood reservoirs were chemically examined on 9 September the previous year, 1931, and both samples were passed as pure. On 11 March 1932, the waters were again examined and some evidence of contamination was found in the sample from Square Wood. These organisms did not, apparently, indicate the presence of sewage but drainage from the land. The sanitary inspector and surveyor had attended to this and the spring supplying the reservoir was sealed. On 6 May the water was reported to be free from pollution.

It was not only the Denby and Cumberworth Council that wanted to clarify a number of misleading points. The outbreak had been reported in *Medical Officer Journal* on 12 November and the following week a letter, penned by P. K. G. Pindar, the Mayor of Scarborough, was published. He wanted, amongst other things, to make it clear that the girl in question had not been on holiday in Scarborough but was a visitor to a village 'some miles' from the town in an area that was not supplied by water form the Scarborough Corporation. The whole episode had, he indicated, come as a surprise to local people of the town as there had been 'no evidence of typhoid contracted in the town'. He concluded by adding that:

As the statement in your paper is likely to prejudice the reputation of Scarborough for the supply of wholesome water, I should be obliged if you would give publicity to this letter equal to that of the somewhat misleading (though I am sure not intentionally misleading) statement in your last issue.[73]

Before we return to Denby Dale it is, perhaps, worth considering this statement for a moment. Clearly, the point is well made and the mayor is likely to be correct when describing the location of the girl's accommodation. That does not mean, of course, that she did not drink the town's water. Given that no residents contracted the disease it is still unlikely that the resort's water was to blame. It may just be worth considering a baffling outbreak in Brighton researched by Sir Arthur Newsholme, a leading authority on state medicine, in 1881. He announced to the sanitary committee there that he had found the cause of such unexplained cases in a previous outbreak that was apparently caused by the eating of oysters. The typhoid bacillus was present in the sewage that twice a day washed over the oyster beds and that the condition in which these oysters lived was 'certainly revolting'.

We shall never know whether there is an outside chance that our visitor enjoyed contaminated oysters in Scarborough but again, if so, why were others not attacked?[74]

The Future of Denby Dale's Water Supplies

The rest of the statement covered the measures detailed in the above sections regarding the closing of the reservoir and the history of the outbreak. It was, incidentally, also reported in the 5 November edition of the *Huddersfield Examiner* that there were six new cases in Malton, a further death there, and three cases at Bailiff Bridge, Brighouse. These cases were not in any way connected with the Denby Dale outbreak. Happily, by the 19 November the papers were able to report that there were no new cases to report in Denby Dale.[75] They did, however, learn that the water from private supplies that many people had chosen to drink was also infected, though not with the typhoid bacteria. It was revealed, following the testing of samples, that the main springs at Heywood Bottom and Hartcliffe Mills were polluted.[76] This 'astonishing revelation' was passed on to the villagers via a notice posted outside the council offices.

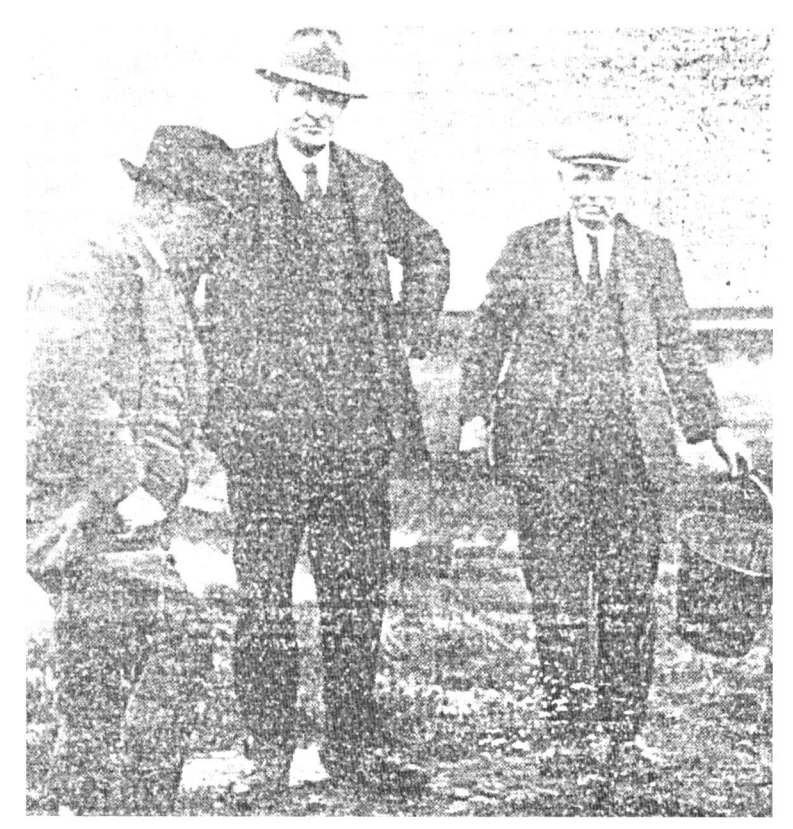

Figure 9:12 Testing the safety of the water at Rusby Wood Reservoir.[77]
(British Library Newspaper Library, Colindale, London.)

This newspaper image shows Council officials testing the inflowing water at nearby Rusby Wood. It is described as showing *Denby Dale Typhoid Epidemic Remedial Work*. The officials' dress and the bucket add a splendid contemporary feel to the picture.

It was also decided, at a further private meeting on 17 November, to engage the services of a firm of Newcastle water engineers to make a survey of all the council's water supplies. The council's minute book of the time provides the information, not reported in the press, that the company employed, after the clerk had received terms from several engineers, was David Balfour and Sons for a fee of thirty guineas (£31.50) plus travelling expenses.[78] This decision had been reached, following a visit to the Ministry of Health in London by the chairman and clerk of the council. After a short but, in many ways, challenging meeting, the tired officials cannot have been thrilled to be greeted at Denby Dale and Cumberworth Railway Station shortly before midnight on Monday, 14 November, by a reporter from the *Holmfirth Express*! A diviner, who had also been engaged to search for new supplies, at the same meeting was able to report that he had made a survey of 121 acres in the Rusby Wood area. He had discovered three new springs that would, in his estimation, yield one hundred thousand gallons of water a day.

The news relating to the water diviner, one B. Tompkins from Norfolk, attracted much interest from the local press, and 'astonished' locals. A reporter from the *Holmfirth Express*, and one assumes other papers, spent some time with him as he went about his task. Up hill and down dale they followed the diviner, a 'heavily built elderly man', and his whitethorn divining rod. As the apex of the stick swerved upwards and backwards Mr. Tompkins had announced that that was 'this is where we are going against the flow of the water'. When he went with the flow the stick, which he held loosely between the middle finger and thumb of each hand, pointed forward. When a spring head was located the rod would, apparently, turn completely over in a whirl. The paper reported this activity without a hint of irony and the nearest the reader came to hearing any views on the matter is a short statement that a 'simple faith in water-diving is not shared by all'![79]

Whatever the views of the people regarding this activity, it was clear that action was needed in relation to future supplies of water for the district. Any future decisions would clearly have the support of the Ministry of Health and it was reported in 'Medical Notes in Parliament' in the *BMJ* in late November that 'steps to were under consideration to procure a water supply free from risk of contamination' in Malton (where there had been eighteen fatalities to date) and Denby Dale. It was also reported by the minister, Sir Hilton Young, that a specifically qualified official of the ministry had investigated the outbreaks and that the source had been traced and eliminated.[80] The council was now able to make plans for the future of Square Wood and any additional supplies as necessary. On 1 December the surveyor reported to the council that a trench across the fields from Rusby Wood had almost been cut, and that pipes to provide an additional supply route had arrived.[81] By 22 December it was announced that the work had been completed.[82] Six weeks later the council resolved that the sanitary inspector, Frederick Greenwood, 'be instructed to take samples of water for testing every two months'[83]

The key meeting with regard to the immediate future of Square Wood was held on 24 May, 1933 when the council met at 10.30 am to receive G.M. McNaughton, the

An Unwelcome Present from Scarborough

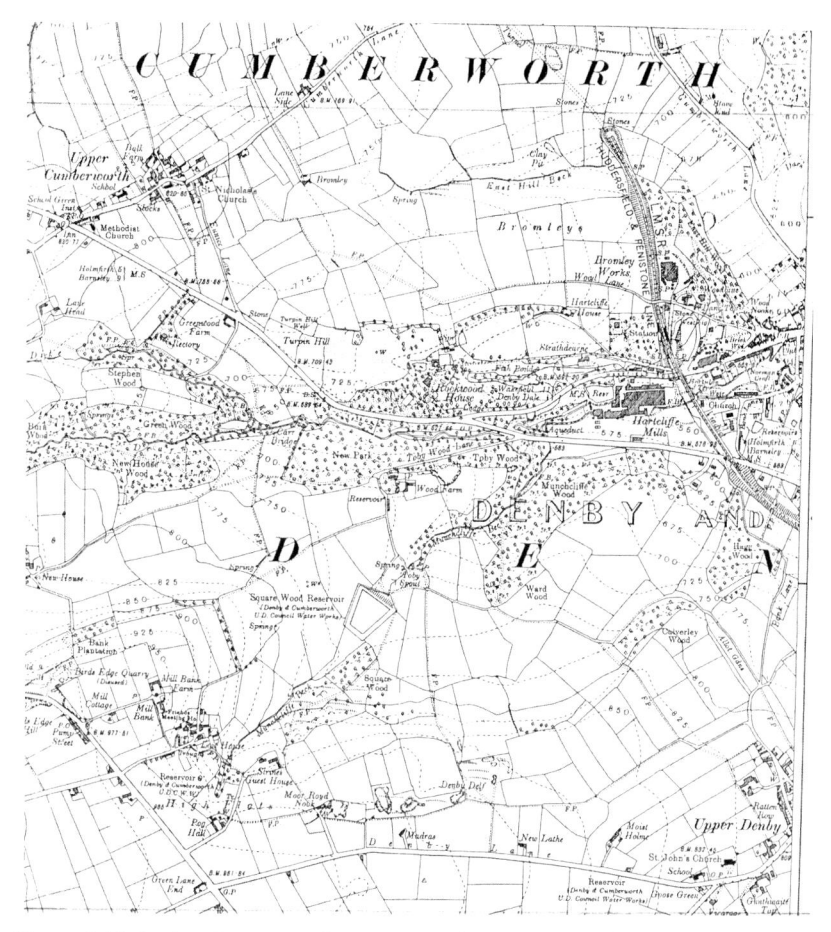

Figure 9:13 Quaker Bottom and Square Wood reservoir in relation to Denby Dale.
(OS Map revised 1929, published 1933. Sheet CCLXXIII NW. Original scale 1:10,560)

Ministry of Health's engineering inspector. By this time Dr. Bleasdell had tendered his resignation, with effect from 31 December of the previous year owing to him leaving the district. The gratitude of the council for his services, especially during the epidemic, was recorded in the minutes. We shall never know whether he gained promotion or resigned because he had simply had enough. Dr. Bleasdell was replaced by his deputy, Dr. G.H. Arnison, who received the same annual salary of £30 as he had.[84] This continued to be a part-time role. The council was still considering returning to the reservoir for the district's water supply after taking 'certain precautions'. This idea was not popular with the local people and at a protest meeting the previous week a resolution had been sent to the Ministry of Health indicting the local people's objection to the scheme. At the meeting the discussion centred around the risk involved in re-opening the reservoir after various remedial schemes were put forward. There are many exchanges reported but what was perhaps the key moment is recorded as follows:

The inspector: *Are you justified in taking the risk?*

Cruel Lives

Councillor Shepley: *No. That is my candid opinion.*
The inspector: *Can you see the Ministry of Health's position in giving sanction to this? Have they the right to risk the lives of people?*
Councillor Shepley: *Not if they are a Ministry of Health.*
Concillor Hinchliffe: *That is what we are here today for, to decide if there is a risk. We don't want to do anything that is not suitable.*

Clearly, alternatives had to be sought, and the meeting then went on to discuss supplies form other sources, including piping water from Broadstones Reservoir and asking the Dewsbury and Heckmondwike Water Board to continue with their help.[85]

It is interesting to read in the minutes the many issues relating to the district's water supply that were discussed prior to, though not directly related to, the epidemic. For example, on 18 August, a few weeks before the outbreak, the surveyor had, ironically, presented an idea to the council regarding additional supplies from Square Wood. The council minute reads as follows:

The surveyor presented his report on a proposal for pumping water from Square Wood to Moistholme reserve in the dry period, in order to augment the present supply for Denby and Toppitt areas. [86]

It is good to report that this scheme was never implemented!

Other examples include investigations into the water supply at the homes of Mrs. Hinchliffe and Mrs. Brown in Polygon Terrace, Denby Dale, in December 1926. The water was from Square Wood and in the first case was 'not fit for use as there are insects in it about a quarter of an inch long'. However, when the samples were taken and tested, there was no evidence of 'living creatures'. At the second home a nurse had reported the water was 'not fit for use'. In 1927 there was concern related to Mrs. Cran of Rockwood Hall who had been in poor health with gastric disorders; and there was a case of enteric fever at Park House, Penistone Road, Birdsedge. In both these cases samples were sent via passenger train, in a special container, to the county laboratory at Wakefield. There was no evidence of pollution reported.[87]

The Final Death is Reported

By mid-November only a few new cases were being reported and the last one appears to be that of a nine-year old girl, Ann Jaques, who was taken to hospital during the second week of November. (Marjorie Jacques - possibly her sister, was one of those excluded from school by Sam Shepley.) It was looking as though no further cases would appear as a few weeks passed without any alarms. However, the microbe had a lethal sting in its tail. On 3 December the Huddersfield Examiner reported that Charles (Clarence in the burial records) Hicks, a single man who lived with his married sister at Exley Gate, Lower Denby had been taken to hospital. He died nine days later.[88] Surprisingly, the epidemic then ended as quietly as it had begun. Yes, there had been a few voices raised in anger as we shall hear, and questions had been asked, not least by those who represented the people.

One such voice was that of the Methodist Minister, Reverend C.A. West, of the Wesley Manse, Denby Dale. In a letter to the paper he expressed outrage at the lack of publicity and was equally annoyed to be told by the chairman of the meeting he attended that 'he had been no help to the meeting and had only criticised'. Reporters from local newspapers had, as we have heard, listened to criticisms and fears from the community. Many houses were not on the water carriage system, a not uncommon situation in both towns and villages at that time, but where this had been installed reporters were informed that water did not enter the main sewerage system but simply ran to earth. In one place, a villager said, sewage ran across the street and 'flows I know not where'. He or she finished by adding the telling comment that: 'You will be doing a great service to the community if you expose the flaws in the sanitary system'.[89]

The sewerage system was, though, little different from those to be found in similar authorities at that time. It was not, however, easy for the members of the council and their employees to live and work in the community. Ron Jackson, who worked for the later Denby Dale Urban District Council as a junior technical assistant for four years from 1956 and as assistant engineer from 1962 to 1964, remembers conversations he had with Frank Horn the waterman. Frank recalled the verbal abuse, including cries of 'murderer', that he and other innocent colleagues received from members of the public.[90]

John Hinchliffe, the chairman, appears to have conducted himself well, as did other

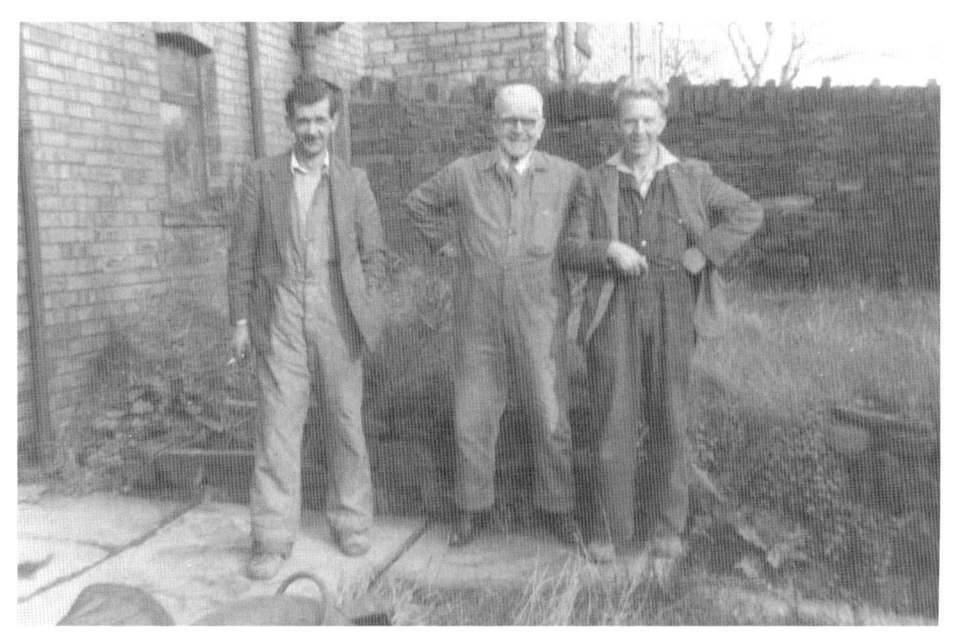

Figure 9:14 Frank Horn (centre) c 1962.
(Ron Jackson collection)

Waterman Frank Horn, shown here to the rear of Denby Dale U.D.C. offices (previously used by Denby and Cumberwoth U.D.C) in Wakefield Road, flanked by colleagues Bill Alderson (left) and, it is believed, Alf George.

Cruel Lives

members of the council, although they must have had many sleepless nights. Their offer to provide each of those infected with a holiday was greatly appreciated, as were their letters of condolence to the families of the victims.[91] The actual number of people who died was twelve. This is the figure also indicated by T.W. Woodhead in his *History of Huddersfield Water Supplies,* although the authors of *A History of Denby Dale Urban District* have the figure as 11.[92]

Walkers who pass the Square Wood reservoir today will see only fishermen as it is no longer used to supply water to the people of Denby Dale. In fact it was never reopened after the epidemic.[93] Those who walk towards the reservoir from, say, Quaker Bottom will, very likely, be unaware of the part it, and the beck, played in the tragedy that occurred some eighty years ago when, in late summer of 1932 a young woman returned from a holiday in Scarborough and was, indirectly and innocently, responsible for the deaths of twelve people. As has already been recorded by others, this was indeed 'the saddest event in the history of Denby Dale'.[94]

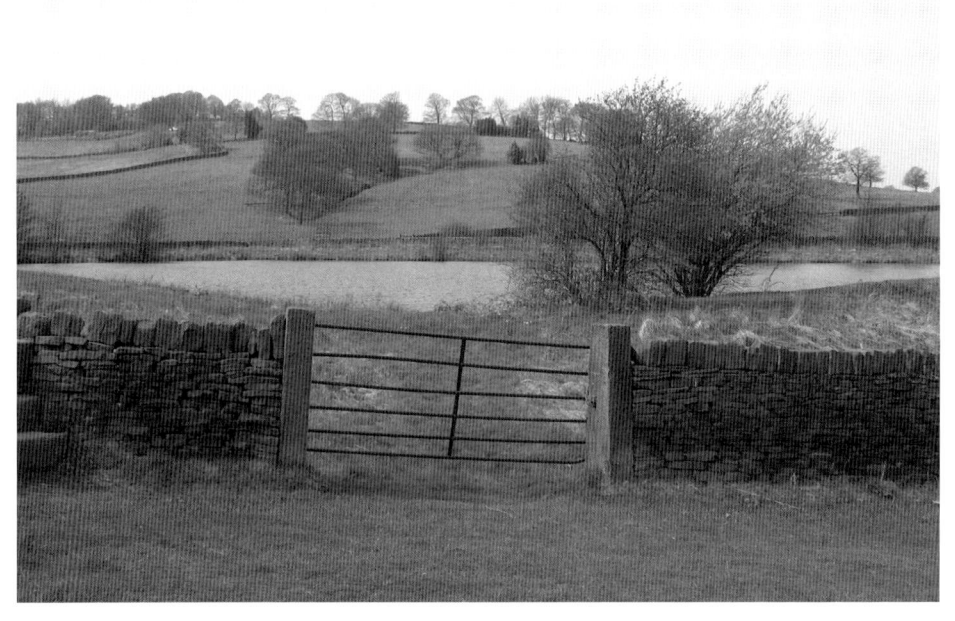

Figure 9:15 Square Wood Reservoir in 2011.

Many who walk past, or fish in, the reservoir today may not be aware of its deadly place in local history.

Appendix

The Twelve Victims

Mrs Ellen Brook* (62)   Leak Hall (Number Two Farm)

Mrs Annie Crossland (61)   Syke House. Lower Denby

Mrs Amy Laundon (44)   Co-operative Terrace.

Lister Stead Peace (72)   Upper Denby.

Thomas Noble (61)   Hartcliffe View.

Ernest Lockwood (31)   Park View.

George Parker (31)   Park View.

Miss Doreen Wood (21)   Co-operative Terrace

Miss Edna Tingle (20)   Penistone (employed in D D)

Arthy Beevers (66)   Smithroyd, Wakefield Road

Fred Wainwright (48)   Hill Side, High Street

Clarence Hicks* (42)   Exley Gate, Lower Denby

This information has been gathered from newspaper reports and burial records. There is much contradictory evidence and where there is doubt I have assumed the burial records to be the more accurate.

*Ellen Brook is listed as Helen Brook in the newspaper, and Clarence Hicks as Charles.

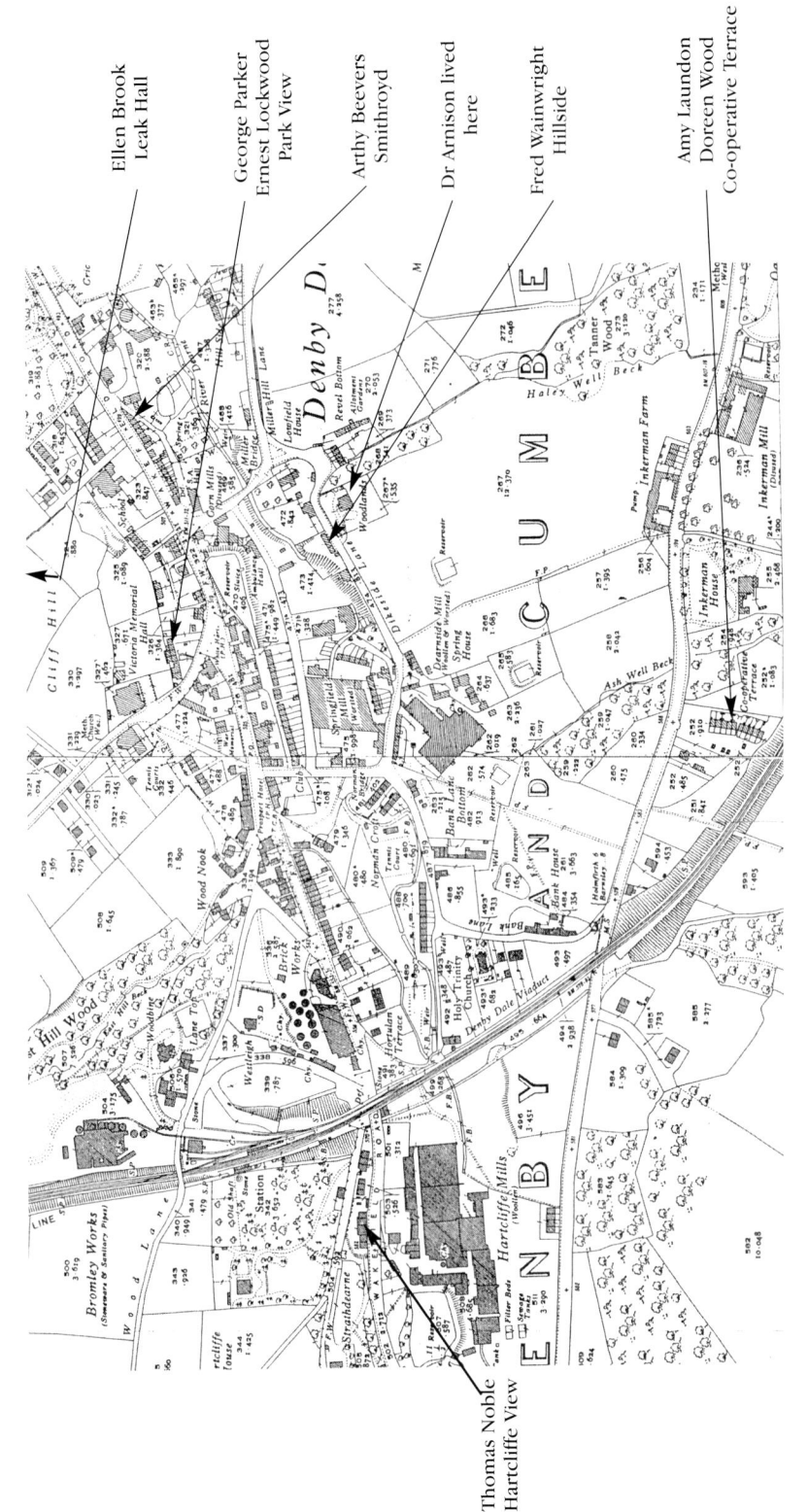

Figure 9.16 The location of the victims' homes in Denby Dale (Ordnance Survey Sheet CCLXVII.3 1933. Original scale 1:2,500)

Eight of the victims lived in what can loosely be termed the central area of Denby Dale. A number of the addresses shown here have since been subsumed into the names of the road that they abut. For example, Park View is now addressed as Cumberworth Lane.

List of Figures

1:1　Bradford from Cliff Quarry, 1873.
1:2　Halifax: North Bridge and Bowling Dyke, 1864.

2:1　South-west Leeds map, 1815.
2:2　St Peter's Church burial register, 1809.
2:3　Marsh Lane Court, 1901.
2:4　Location map: Marsh Lane Court.

3:1　Leeds from Rope-Hill, c1840.
3:2　The Boot and Shoe Yard location.
3:3　Robert Baker's grave
3:4　The Cherry Tree Yard, 1901.
3:5　The location of the Cherry Tree Yard.
3:6　St. Peter's Church burial register, June 1832
3:7　St. Peter's Church burial register, August 1832.
3:8　Robert Baker.
3:9　Sanitary map of Leeds, 1839.

4:1　Goulden's Square, Leeds, 1901.
4:2　Location map: Slack, Hebden Bridge and Heptonstall
4:3　1851 census return Slack, 1851
4:4　Lumb Mills c1900.
4:5　Map of Slack, 1848.

5:1　Archibald Tait.
5:2　Halifax from Beacon Hill. Late nineteenth century.
5:3　Location of Roils Head Farm.
5:4　1881 census return.
5:5　Location map: Hopwood Lane.
5:6　Hopwood Lane map detail.
5:7　St Paul's School log book, 1881.
5:8　Halifax c1890.

6:1　The location of the Spen Valley towns.
6:2　Cleckheaton, 1905.
6:3　1881 census return.
6:4　Broomfield Mills: entrance arch, 2006
6:5　Elymas Wadsworth.
6:6　The Revd. E.W. Easton
6:7　Edward Wadsworth.
6:8　Cleckheaton, 1914.

7:1　Vine Farm, Clifton. 1950s.
7:2　Smallpox patient.
7:3　Savile Lane, Clifton. 1950s.
7:4　Location map, Savile Lane. 1907.

7:5   Clifton School logbook, 1892.
7:6   Brighouse 1894.
7:7   Brighouse town centre map, 1892.
7:8   The Brighouse News, 1892.
7:9   1891 Census return, Police Street.
7:10 Kiln Fold, c1904.
7:11 Eli Walton's death certificate.
7:12 Brighouse Town centre c1904
7:13 1891 Census return, Firth Street.
7:14 Public notice, May 1892.
7:15 Advertisement, Brighouse Echo,1892.
7:16 Edward Jenner.
7:17 Clifton Hospital building, 2002.
7:18 Clifton Hospital site plan.

8:1   Central Bradford c1890
8:2   South Bradford map, c 1900.
8:3   St. Stephen's School: Immediate environs.
8:4   St. Stephen's school: Log book entries
8:5   MOH letter to parents.
8:6   St. Stephen's School: original building.

9:1   Location map. Denby Dale.
9:2   Kitty Robson c 1931.
9:3   Green Hollows, 2012.
9:4   Quaker Bottom map, 1933.
9:5   Denby Dale from the west, c1922
9:6   Denby Dale School log book, 1932.
9:7   The Huddersfield Examiner 1932
9:8   The Wood, Parker and Lockwood family tree.
9:9   Doreen Wood c1929.
9:10 Sketch map: How contamination of Square Wood Reservoir occurred.
9:11 Wakefield Road, Denby Dale, 1928.
9:12 Testing the water at Rusby Wood, 1932
9:13 Denby Dale in relation to Square Wood, 1933.
9:14 Frank Horn, c1962.
9:15 Square Wood Reservoir, 2011.

List of Tables

1:1 Population Growth, 1801 -1851.
1:2 Average age of death 1842.
1:3 Prevalent disease deaths 1840 – 1910.

2:1 Funerals: St, Peter's Church, Leeds, 1809.
2:2 Measles victims' ages, 1809.

3:1 Age and sex distribution of cholera mortality, Leeds 1832.

4:1 Ages of Slack residents, 1844.
4:2 Ages of fever cases, 1844.

5:1 Scarlet fever cases reported, 1880-81.
5:2 Distibution of Robert Bell's milk.
5:3 Milk distribution in thirteen streets.

6:1 Death notices March - August 1881.
6:2 Age groups of victims.
6:3 Liversedge Local Board mortality rates 1880-91.

7:1 Cases and deaths 1892-93
7:2 Vaccinated and unvaccinated cases survival figures.

8:1 Diphtheria mortality Bradford, 1900- 04.
8:2 Monthly deaths, 1904.
8:3 Victims' ages.

9:1 Denby Dale hospital lists November, 1932.

Notes

Chapter One: The Epidemic Streets

1. S. Halliday, *The Great Filth*, (Sutton Publishing, 2007), pp. 18-19.
2. A.S. Wohl, *Endangered Lives*, (J.M. Dent, & Sons Ltd, 1984), p. 4.
3. Information gathered from day course at Bradford University, 26 April, 2008.
4. J. Burnett, *A Social History of Housing: 1815-1985*, (2nd edition, Methuen, 1986)
5. Information from day course at Bradford University. 26 April, 2008.
6. J. Burnett, (1986), p. 10.
7. B.R. Mitchell, *Abstract of British Historical Statistics*, (Cambridge University Press, 1988), pp. 24-27.
8. J. Burnett, (1986), p.10.
9. *ibid*, p.13.
10. The *Leeds Intelligencer*, 14 June 1832.
11. J. Burnett, (1986), p.11.
12. J. Hole, *The Homes of the Working Classes*, (1866), p. 45.
13. S. Pierson, 'The Way Out', in H.J. Dyas and M. Wolff, *The Victorian City: Images and Realities, Volume 2*, (Routledge and Kegan Paul 1973), p. 873.
14. E. Gauldie, *Cruel Habitations*, (George Allen and Unwin, 1974), p. 188.
15. S. Halliday, (2007), p. 20.
16. A.S. Wohl, (1984), p. 12.
17. *ibid*, p. 11.
18. A. Briggs, *Victorian Cities*, (Pelican Books, 1968).
19. E. Chadwick, *Report on the Sanitary Condition of the Labouring Population of Great Britain*, 1842, edited M.W. Flinn, (Edinburgh, 1965), p. 244.
20. A.S. Wohl, (1986), p.11.
21. *ibid*, pp. 13-14.
22. E. Chadwick, (1842), p. 223.
23. *ibid*, p. 224.
24. J. Burnett, (1986), p. 104.
25. E.E. Lampard, 'The Urbanizing World' in H.J. Dyas, and M.Wolff, *The Victorian City: Images and Realities*, Volume 1, (Routledge and Kegan Paul, 1973), p. 20.
26. S. Halliday, (2007), p. 21.
27. S.R. Whitehead, *The Brontes' Haworth* (Ashmount Press, 2006) p. 81.
28. G. Rosen, 'Disease, Debility and Death', in H.J. Dyas, and M. Wolff, (1973) p.626.
29. *ibid*, p. 625.
30. *ibid*, p. 659.
31. A.S. Wohl, 'Unfit for Human Habitation', in H.J. Dyas, and M. Wolff, (1973), p.611.
32. *ibid*, p. 612.
33. *ibid*, p. 611.
34. T. Hunt, *National Trust Magazine*, Spring 2010, p. 20.
35. *ibid*, p. 613.
36. J. Hole, (1866), p. 3.

37 F. Engels, *The Conditions of the Working Class in England,* 1845, Leipzig; 1892, London, (Panther Books,1969), p. 61.
38 *ibid,* pp. 74-75.
39 J. Hole, (1866), p. 134.
40 A.S. Wohl, (1986), p. 235.
41 J. Hole, (1866), p. 48 quoting J. Ruskin.
42 M. Bull: *Calderdale Companion* website. 2011. (www.calderdalecompanion.co.uk)
43 *Report of the Leeds Board of Health*, 1833, (Printed by Hernaman and Perring at the Intelligencer Office, Leeds,1833), pp.21-27
44 E. Gaskell, *Mary Barton,* 1848, (Oxford University Press, 2006), p. 58.
45 C. Dickens, *Little Dorrit,* 1855-57, (Odhams Press,1930), p.39.
46 A.S. Wohl, (1986), p. 286.
47 C. Dickens, *Hard Times,* 1854, (Odhams Press,1930), p. 24.
48 W. Ranger, *Preliminary Inquiry as to the Sewerage, Drainage and Supply of Water of Halifax,* (Publisher unknown, 1851), p. 40.
49 E. Chadwick, (1842).
50 S. Halliday, (2007), p. 141.
51 E. Chadwick, (1842), p. 190.
52 *ibid,* p. 193.
53 M. Beresford, *East End, West End*, (The Thorseby Society, 1988), p. 417.
54 *ibid,* p. 418.
55 E.R. Dewsnap, quoted by E.E. Lampard, 1973, p. 22.
56 M. Beresford, (1988), p. 205.
57 J. Burnett, (1986), p. 70.
58 *Halifax MOH Report*, 1876, p. 11.
59 W. Ranger, (1851), p. 18.
60 *ibid,* p. 77.
61 M. Beresford, (1988), p. 204.
62 A.S. Wohl, (1986), p. 43.
63 S. Halliday, (2007), p. 58.
64 A. Hardy, *The Epidemic Streets* (Oxford University Press, 1993), p. 211.
65 J.F. Churchill, *Consumption and Tuberculosis,* (Longman, Green, 1875) Introduction.
66 D.H. Crawford, *Deadly Companions,* (Oxford University Press, 2009), p.159.
67 A. Hardy, (1993), pp. 211-266 & S. Halliday, (2007), p. 86.

Chapter Two: The Fatal Effects of a Malady

1 A.S. Wohl, *Endangered Lives,* (Methuen, 1983), p. 288.
2 *Report on an Occurrence of Measles in Epidemic Form,* Borough of Leeds, 1891.
3 D.H. Crawford, *Deadly Companions,* (Oxford University Press, 2007), p. 63.
4 News items and articles in the *Daily Telegraph Magazine*, 2007; *The Times*, 14 July, 2010 & *The Sunday Times,* 17 April, 2011.
5 F.B. Smith, *The People's Health,* (Weidenfield & Nicolson, 1990), pp. 142-3.
6 A. Hardy, *The Epidemic Streets,* (Clarendon Press, 1993), p. 9.

7. R. Woods & N. Shelton, *An Atlas of Victorian Mortality,* (Liverpool University Press, 2007), p. 63.
8. C. Creighton, *A History of Epidemics in Great Britain*, Vol. 2 (Cambridge University Press, 1894; Reprinted Frank Cass, 1965) p. 674.
9. Lightcliffe National School logbooks, (Lightcliffe C. E. Primary School).
10. D.H. Crawford, (2007), p. 63.
11. F.B. Smith, (1990), p. 147.
12. A.S. Wohl, (1983), p. 135 and F.B. Smith, 1990, p. 146.
13. B.A.Whitelegge,1892, Measles Epidemics Major & Minor in *Transactions of the Epidemiological Society, of London,* 1892, p. 45.
14. M. Dobson, *Disease,* (Quercus, 2007), pp. 144-5.
15. *Pears Cyclopaedia,* (Pears,1898), p. 692.
16. *ibid*, p. 714.
17. R. Woods & N. Shelton, (1997), p. 144.
18. B.A. Whitelegge, (1892), p. 37.
19. F.B. Smith, (1990), pp. 65-9.
20. *ibid*, pp. 144-5.
21. The *Leeds Mercury*, 10 June, 1809.
22. Leeds Parish Church Burial Register, 1809. (West Yorkshire Archive Service [WYAS], Leeds, Ref: RDP68/3/B/7)
23. I am grateful to the Thoresby Society for this information.
24. B.A. Whitelegge, (1892), p. 45.
25. Borough of Leeds, 1891.
26. *ibid*.
27. B.A. Whitelegge, (1892), p. 45.
28. I am grateful to David Thornton of the Thoresby Society, Leeds, for drawing my attention to these figures.
29. *Report of the Health and Sanitary Administration of the City for the Year 1918* (William Angus, MOH, Leeds, 1918).
30. B.A. Whitelegge, (1892), p. 53.

Chapter Three: A Tidal wave of Disease

1. The *Leeds Intelligencer*, 5 April 1832.
2. K. Hoole, *A Regional History of the Railways of Great Britain Volume 4: The North East*, (David and Charles, 1965), pp.29 and 39.
3. The *Leeds Intelligencer*, 10 May 1832.
4. M. Durey, *The Return of the Plague: British Society and the Cholera, 1831-32*, (Gill and MacMillan, 1979), p. 31.
5. D.V. Smith, *The First Asiatic Cholera Epidemic in Leeds, 1832*, (Leeds, 1982), p. 4. A copy of this unpublished work is retained in Leeds Central Library.
6. The *Leeds Intelligencer,* 14 April 1832.
7. C.F. Brockington, *Public Health in the Nineteenth Century*, (E. and S. Livingstone) p. 76.
8. R.J. Morris, *Cholera 1832,* (Croom Helm), p. 11.
9. Smith (1982), p. 4.
10. The *Leeds Mercury*, 9 June 1832.

Notes

[11] The *Leeds Intelligencer*, 8 December 1831.
[12] A.S. Wohl, *Endangered Lives,* (Methuen,1983), pp. 118-19 & M. Holland, G. Gill & S. Burrell, *Cholera and Conflict,* Medical Museum Publishing, (2009), pp. 1-2.
[13] Durey (1979), p. 34.
[14] D. Hill, *Turner and Leeds: Images of Industry,* (Northern Arts, 2008)
[15] The *Leeds Mercury*, 10 May 1832.
[16] Durey (1979), p. 34.
[17] E.A. Underwood, (1935), 'A History of the 1832 Cholera Epidemic in Yorkshire', *Proceedings of the Royal Society of Medicine* 1935, p. 606.
[18] The *Leeds Intelligencer*, 2 June 1832.
[19] M.D. Beresford, *East End, West End: The Face of Leeds during Urbanisation,* (The Thoresby Society Leeds, 1988), p. 392.
[20] *Report of the Leeds Board of Health, 1833.* Printed by Hernaman and Perring at the Intelligencer Office, Leeds, 1833, p. 7.
[21] Beresford, (1988), p. 392.
[22] Smith, (1982), p. 13.
[23] *ibid.*
[24] The *Leeds Intelligencer*, 14 June 1832.
[25] *ibid.*
[26] M.D. Beresford, 'The Back-to-Back House in Leeds, 1787-1937' in S.D. Chapman, *A History of Working Class Housing,* (David and Charles, 1971), p. 100.
[27] Beresford (1988), p. 82.
[28] *ibid*, p. 47 and p. 122, footnote 11.
[29] M.D. Beresford, 'The Face of Leeds' in Fraser, D., *A History of Modern Leeds,* (Manchester University Press, 1980), pp. 76 & 287.
[30] *ibid*, p.75. From an original in Leeds City Archives, LCEng.Box10.
[31] J.A. Burnett, 'A Social History of Housing, 1815-1985', (Methuen, 1978), p. 9.
[32] N. Longmate, *King Cholera: The Biography of a Disease,* (David and Charles, Newton Abbot, 1966), p. 97.
[33] The *Leeds Mercury*, 9 June 1832.
[34] *Report of the Leeds Board of Health*, 1833, p. 13.
[35] 'Robert Baker, CB', *The British Medical Journal,* 6 March 1880, p. 383 and W.R. Lee 'Robert Baker: The First Doctor in the Factory Department, Part 1.1803-1858 *British Journal of Industrial Medicine,* 1964, vol. 21, pp. 85-90. I am grateful to Alan Humphries, Librarian at the Thackray Medical Museum, Leeds for his help in locating a number of references relating to Robert Baker.
[36] The *Leeds Intelligencer*, 18 March 1826.
[37] 'Robert Baker, CB' (1880), p. 383 and 'Robert Baker: The First Doctor in the Factory Department, (1964), pp. 85-90.
[38] R. Baker, 'On the State and Condition of the Town of Leeds in the West Riding of the County of York', (Leeds, 1842), quoted in S. Barnard, *To Prove I'm Not Forgot,* (Manchester University Press, 1990), p. 23.
[39] E. Chadwick, *Report on the Sanitary Condition of the Labouring Population of Great Britain,* 1842. Edited, M.W. Flinn, (Edinburgh, 1965), p. 103.
[40] The *British Medical Journal*, 6 March, 1880, p. 383.
[41] *ibid.*

[42] Underwood (1935), p. 615.
[43] Photograph reproduced with permission of Leeds City Library and Information Services. Book reference: LQ331.833. *Photographs of slum clearance from Leeds City Engineer's Department*. Vol.5. Leodis website collection ref 20021010-15305727.
[44] Beresford, (1971), p. 110.
[45] N. Longmate, (1966), p. 97.
[46] S. Burrell, S. and G.V. Gill, 'The British Cholera Riots of 1832' in *Swing Unmasked - the Agricultural Riots of 1830-1832 and their Wider Implications*, Ed. Holland, M., (FACHRS Publications, Milton Keynes, 2005) p. 202.
[47] S. Johnson, *The Ghost Map*, (Allen Lane, 2006), pp. 191-228.
[48] Underwood, (1935), p. 605.
[49] Smith, (1982), p. 25.
[50] *Report to the Leeds Board of Health, 1833*, p. 13.
[51] Underwood, (1935), p. 614.
[52] *ibid*.
[53] *Report to the Leeds Board of Health*, 1833, p. 7.
[54] *ibid*, p. 8.
[55] *ibid*, p. 10.
[56] *ibid*, p. 12.
[57] *ibid*, p. 19.
[58] Smith (1982) p. 24.
[59] Beresford (1988), p. 391.
[60] The *Leeds Mercury,* 12 November 1831.
[61] M. Durey, *The First Spasmodic Cholera Epidemic in York,* (Borthwick Institute Paper 48) 1974, p. 13.
[62] S.T. Anning. *The History of Medicine in Leeds,* (Leeds, 1980), p. 167.
[63] A History of the Leeds School of Medicine, (Leeds, 1982), p. 8.
[64] The *Lancet,* Volume 21,1832, p. 672.
[65] *Report to the Leeds Board of Health, 1833*, p. 10.
[66] Durey, (1974), p. 13.
[67] The *Leeds Mercury,* 25 August 1832.
[68] Brockington (1965), p. 67.
[69] The *Leeds Mercury,* 18 August 1832.
[70] J. Kay, The Moral and Physical Conditions of the working Classes Employed in the Cotton Manufacture of Manchester, (Manchester),1832, p. 11.
[71] I am grateful to Mrs. Ann Clark, Parish Warden, Leeds Parish Church, and the Revd. Peter Sutcliffe former Vicar of St. Matthew's, Lightcliffe, for information in relation to the interpretation of the clergy titles.
[72] *ibid*.
[73] Beresford (1988), p. 389.
[74] *ibid*.
[75] S. Barnard, *To Prove I'm Not Forgot: Living and Dying in a Victorian City,* (Manchester University Press, (1990), pp.4 & 10.
[76] *ibid*, p.32.
[77] St. Peter's Parish Church, Leeds, *Burial Records 1832-34,* West Yorkshire Archive Service, Ref: RDP68/3B/7
[78] Underwood, (1935), p. 8.

Notes

[79] *Report to the Leeds Board of Health*, (1833), p. 12.
[80] The *Lancet,* volume, 22, 1832, p. 671.
[81] *Celebrating 175 years,* (Leeds School of Medicine Programme, 2006).
[82] Thackrah, C.T., *Cholera, its Character and Treatment* (J. Baines & Co., Leeds, 1832) pp. 41-45.
[83] Leeds School of Medicine: *Celebrating 175 years*. Programme, autumn, 2006.
[84] The *Leeds Mercury*, 16 June 1832.
[85] *ibid.*
[86] The *Leeds Intelligencer*, 9 August 1832.
[87] *ibid,* 2 August 1832.
[88] The *Leeds Mercury*, 11 June 1832.
[89] The *Leeds Mercury*, 1 December 1831.
[90] *ibid,* 29 October 1831.
[91] Smith (1832), p. 26.
[92] Information gleaned from the Leeds Historical Society Exhibition, *The Borough of Leeds, 1207-2007,* (June, 2007)
[93] F. Engels, *The Condition of the Working Class in England* (1892, as reprinted 1976), p. 326.
[94] The *Leeds Mercury*, 29 October 1831.
[95] The *Leeds Intelligencer*, 24 November 1831.
[96] Johnson, S., (2006), p. 104.
[97] The *Leeds Intelligencer*, 24 November 1831.
[98] Correspondence and information from the Thackray Medical Museum quoted by Fernando, M. and Puntis, J. in *Yorkshire Medicine,* Spring 2001, p. 43.
[99] Thackrah, C.T., 1832, p. 60.
[100] The *Leeds Intelligencer*, 26 March 1832.
[101] Durey, (1979), p. 150.
[102] *ibid,* pp. 21-23.
[103] Anning, (1980), p. 138.
[104] Quoted in *Robert Baker, CB.,* BMJ, 1880, p. 86.
[105] The *Leeds Intelligencer*, 18 March 1826.
[106] The *Leeds Intelligencer*, 5 April 1832.
[107] *ibid.*
[108] The *Leeds Intelligencer*, 29 March 1832.
[109] Hemp, A., *Briggate:A History in Pictures,*(Leeds City Library, Leeds, 1988), p. 18
[110] Anning (1980), page 139, quoting Mayhall, J., *The Annals of Yorkshire,* (Leeds,1861), p. 382.
[111] *The Times*, 11 February 1832.
[112] Durey (1982), p. 169
[113] The *Leeds Intelligencer*, 14 June 1832.
[114] The *Leeds Mercury*, 28 April 1832.
[115] The *Leeds Intelligencer*, 14 June, 1832.
[116] Smith, (1982), p. 15.
[117] Barnard (1990), p. 1.
[118] S.T. Anning, and W.K.J. Walls, *A History of the Leeds Medical School, 1831-1981,* (Leeds,1982), pp. 71-72. W. R. Lee, *Robert Baker: The First Doctor in the Factory Department,* Part 1, p. 86; Part 2, p. 168.

[119] The *Leeds Intelligencer*, 14 June 1832.
[120] *ibid*.
[121] The *Leeds Mercury*, 9 June 1832.
[122] The *Leeds Intelligencer*, 14 June 1832.
[123] *ibid*, 10 June, 1832, and Smith, D.V., 1982, p. 16.
[124] Smith, (1982), p. 14.
[125] The *Leeds Intelligencer*, 14 June 1832.
[126] Smith (1982), p. 22.
[127] Underwood, (1935), p. 604.
[128] Wohl, (1983), p. 118.
[129] Smith, (1982), p. 30.
[130] Beresford, (1988), p. 397.
[131] Barnard, (1990), p. 23.
[132] Beresford, (1988), p. 392.
[133] E. Chadwick, (1842), *The Sanitary Condition of the Labouring Population of Great Britain*, Map between pages 160-61. Reproduced from original copy of book in Thackray Medical Museum.
[134] E. Chadwick, (1842), Ed. Flinn, M.W., (Edinburgh University Press, Edinburgh, 1965), page 51
[135] *ibid*, p. 24.
[136] Anning (1980), p. 6.
[137] *ibid*, p. 73.
[138] *ibid*.
[139] Burrell, S. and Gill, G., 'The Liverpool Cholera Epidemic of 1832' and Anatomical Dissection In *Journal of History of Medicine and Allied Sciences*, (2005) volume 60, number 4, p. 498.
[140] R.J. Morris, (1976), p. 117.
[141] The *Leeds Intelligencer*, 10 November 1831.
[142] A. Briggs, *Victorian Cities*, (1963), p. 149.

Chapter Four: An Aggravated Calamity

[1] R. Howard, *History of the Typhus of Heptonstall-Slack*, (W. Garforth, Hebden Bridge, 1844) Preface.
[2] A.S. Wohl, *Endangered Lives*, (Methuen, 1984), pp. 125-6.
[3] M. Dobson, *Disease*, (Quercus, 2007), pp. 36-8.
[4] D.H. Crawford, *Deadly Companions*, (Oxford University Press, 2009) p. 152.
[5] A. Hardy, *The Epidemic Streets*, (Clarendon Press, 1993), pp. 152-3.
[6] *ibid*, pp. 193 and 210.
[7] F.F. Cartwright, *Disease and History*, (Rupert Hart-Davis, 1972), pp. 89, 100-1.
[8] C. Creighton, *A History of Epidemics in Britain: Volume 2*, (Cambridge University Press, 1894; Frank Cass reprint, 1965), p. 160.
[9] H. Kennally, Famine, Typhus & the Poor Law: Irish Families in Leeds in *Publications of the Thoresby Society*, Second Series, Volume 20 (2010), p. 62-3.
[10] *ibid*, p. 65.
[11] *ibid*, p. 70.
[12] *ibid*, pp. 68 & 70.

[13] Creighton, (1894, 1965), p. 207.
[14] G. Figures, 'Typhus, Two Windows and a Gold Chain' in *Publications of the Thoresby Society*. Second Series, Volume 20 (2010) pp. 75-85.
[15] Howard, *History of the Typhus of Heponstall-Slack,* (W Garforth, Hebden Bridge, 1844)
[16] *ibid*, p. iv.
[17] Howard, (1844), p. 68.
[18] *ibid*, p. 15.
[19] *ibid*, p. 57.
[20] I am grateful to Justine Wyatt for this information.
[21] I. Bailey, 'Sacrificed at the Shrine of Avarice?' In *Pennine Perspectives: Aspects of the History of Midgley,* Ed. I. Bailey, D. Cant, A. Petford, N. Smith. (Midgley Books, 2007), p.221.
[22] 1851 census returns.
[23] Bailey, (2007), p. 222.
[24] J. Wyatt, (co-ordinator) *Power in the Landscape* (Hebden Bridge Alternative Technology Centre, 2007), p. 8.
[25] *ibid* p. 19.
[26] Howard, (1844), p. 12.
[27] *ibid.* ,pp. 12-13.
[28] Howard, (1944), p 69.
[29] *ibid*, pp. 42-43, 48.
[30] I am grateful for the advice given here by Dr. Steven Chambers, Professor Geoff Gill and Dr. Alan Greenwood.
[31] Taken from the General Practitioners' notebook: iGP. (www.gpnotebook.co.uk)

Chapter Five: A Farmer, a Hired Man and a Milk Round

[1] H.H. Scott, *Some Notable Epidemics*, Edward Arnold, (1934), p. 165.
[2] F.B. Smith, *The People's Health*, (Wiedenfeld & Nicolson, 1990), p. 136.
[3] A.S. Wohl, *Endangered Lives*, (Methuen 1984), p. 129.
[4] The *British Medical Journal (BMJ)*, 6 May, 1933, p. 806.
[5] A. Hardy, *The Epidemic Streets*, (Clarendon Press, 1993), pp. 59 & 65.
[6] The *Halifax Guardian*, 8 January 1881.
[7] C. Creighton, *A History of Epidemics in Britain, Volume 2*, (Cambridge University Press, 1894 Frank Cass reprint, 1965), pp. 726-27.
[8] J.G. Washington, 'Isolation Hospitals in Halifax', in *Transactions of the Halifax Antiquarian Society,* Volume 7 (New Series), 1999, p. 122.
[9] *Report of the Medical Officer of Health (MOH)*, 1899, Bradford p. 28
[10] C. Clark, & R. Davison, *In Loving Memory*: *The Story of Undercliffe Cemetery,* (Sutton Publishing), p. 85.
[11] J. Paxman, *The Victorians,* BBC Books, (2009), p. 147 and on-line 1861 census return.
[12] The *British Medical Journal*, 22 January, 1881, p. 130.
[13] *Report of the MOH*, 31 December 1881, Borough of Halifax, p. 3.
[14] *ibid*, p. 6.
[15] *BMJ*, 12 February 1881, p. 255.

[16] *ibid*, 22 January 1881, p. 130.
[17] *ibid*, 12 February 1881, p. 242.
[18] A. Betteridge and D. Bridge, *Maps and Views of Old Halifax*, (Ryburn Publishing, 1991).
[19] B. Wadsworth, *Edward Wadsworth: A Painter's Life*, (Michael Russell, 1989), p. 89. A number of versions of this story exist and some indicate, as Barbara Wadsworth does, that Edward Wadsworth prefaced his comment with 'it's beautiful'.
[20] J.M. Eyler, *Sir Arthur Newsholme and State Medicine, 1885-1935*, (Cambridge UP, 1997), p. 127.
[21] Creighton, C, p. 734.
[22] *BMJ*, 12 February 1881, p. 255.
[23] Scott, (1934), p.168.
[24] The *Halifax Guardian*, 8 January 1881, p. 4.
[25] *ibid*.
[26] Scott, (1934), p. 169.
[27] *ibid*, p.171
[28] The *Halifax Guardian*, 8 January 1881, p. 4.
[29] *MOH Report*, Halifax, p. 7.
[30] *ibid*.
[31] Scott, (1934), p. 168.
[32] The *Halifax Courier*, 15 January 1881.
[33] *ibid*, 15 January, 1881
[34] The *Halifax Courier*, 15 January 1881.
[35] *ibid* and the *Halifax Guardian*, 15 January 1881.
[36] The *Halifax Guardian*, 29 January 1881.
[37] The *Halifax Courier*, 29 January 1881. The *Halifax Guardian* reported on the same day that the cases numbered 337 - two more of scarlet fever.
[38] The *Halifax Guardian*, 22 January 1881.
[39] *Kelly's Directory*, Kelly and Co., 1881, p. 39
[40] St. Paul's, King Cross, burial records, 1881, pp. 259-60, Huddersfield Local Studies Library.
[41] Information from Ancestry.co.uk.
[42] Scott, (1934), p. 172.
[43] The *Halifax Courier* and The *Halifax Guardian* 15 January 1881.
[44] The *Halifax Courier*, 15 January 1881.
[45] *ibid*.
[46] The *Halifax Guardian*, 22 January 1881.
[47] West Yorkshire Archive Service (WYAS: Calderdale) OR/ED 240a (i)
[48] *ibid*, OR/ED 248 (i &iii).
[49] *ibid*, OR/ED 245c (i).
[50] *ibid*, OR/ED 245a (i).
[51] J. Brooke, *When Panic Seized the Town*, Rastrick High School, 2003, p. 16.
[52] WYAS: Calderdale, OR/ED 248 (i &iii)
[53] S.G. Waring, *The Sanitary drainage of Houses and Towns*, (Houghton & Osgood, 1879), pp. 265-70
[54] The *Halifax Courier* and the *Halifax Guardian*, 15 January 1881.
[55] The *Leeds Mercury*, 31 January 1881.

56 The *Halifax Courier*, 15 January 1881.
57 The *Halifax Guardian*, 22 January 1881.
58 The *Halifax Courier*, 1 February 1881.
59 Washington, (1999), p. 121 & 126. [for a detailed history of the development of Stoney Royd and other Halifax Isolation Hospitals see J.G. Washington's paper in Transactions of the Halifax Antiquarian Society, Volume 7 (New series), pp.117-136].
60 Smith, (1990), p139.
61 The *Leeds Mercury*, 23 January 1881.
62 The *Halifax Courier*, 1 February 1881.
63 *Sedbergh Historian*, Volume V, no. 5, p. 32.
64 *BMJ*, 12 February 1881, p. 255
65 Brooke, (2003), p. 34.
66 The *Halifax Guardian*, 29 January 1881.
67 A. Betteridge et al, *Calderdale Architecture and History*, (Ryburn Publishing, 1988), Images 80-83.
68 BMJ, 19 February, 1881.
69 The *Halifax Guardian*, 12 February 1881.
70 *BMJ*, 19 February 1881.
71 Scott, (1934), p.171.
72 *ibid*, p. 169.
73 *Report of the MOH*, Borough of Halifax 31 December, 1881, pp. 6.
74 Scott, (1934), p. 170.
75 *ibid*, p.171.
76 The *Leeds Mercury*, 26 April 1881.
77 Scott, (1934), pp. 169-171.
78 I am grateful to Mrs. Mavis Armitage and Dr. Alan Greenwood for this information.
79 C.L. Scamman. Presented at a joint session of American Public Health Association, *1929*. In *American Journal of Public Health*, pp. 1139-1146.
80 R. Watson, *British Medical Journal, 12 June 1937*, pp. 1189-1193.
81 *ibid*, pp.1192-3.
82 Scammon, (1929), p. 1345.
83 J.M. Eyler, (1997), p. 139.
84 *Report of the MOH*, Borough of Halifax 31 December, 1881, pp. 5-9
85 *ibid*, 1882, p. 4.
86 *ibid*, and list of tables, 1881.

Chapter Six: A Memorable Visitation

1 The *Cleckheaton and Spen Valley Guardian*, 5 June 1891.
2 G. M. Howe, *Man, Environment and Disease in Britain*, (David and Charles, 1972), p. 188.
3 D.H. Crawford, *Deadly Companions*, (Oxford University Press, 2007) p. 205.
4 M. Honigsbaum, *Living with Enza*, (Macmillan, 2009) p.15.
5 M. Dobson, *Disease*, (Quercus, 2007) p.172.
6 A.H. Gale, *Epidemic Diseases*, (Penguin/Pelican, 1959) p. 44.

[7] F.B. Smith, *The People's Health,* (Weidenfeld and Nicolson, 1990) p. 323.
[8] Dobson, (2007), p. 175.
[9] K.D. Patterson, *Pandemic Influenza 1700-1900,* (Rowman and Littlefield, 1986) p. 51.
[10] Smith, (1990), p. 324.
[11] Honigsbaum, (2009) p. 15.
[12] *ibid.*
[13] J. Nicolson, 'Flu in 1918-19', *Daily Telegraph* feature, 11 November 2009.
[14] Honigsbaum, (2009), p.viii.
[15] *ibid,* p. 15.
[16] T.W. Thompson, *The Spen Valley: A Local History,* (Senior and Co. Ltd, The Heckmondwike Herald, 1925), p. 250-51.
[17] The *Cleckheaton and Spen Valley Guardian*, 1 May 1891.
[18] The *British Medical Journal*, 25 April 1891, p. 929.
[19] *ibid,* 8 August 1891, p. 307.
[20] The *Cleckheaton and Spen Valley Guardian*, 1 May 1891.
[21] *ibid.*
[22] The *Dewsbury Reporter*, 2 May 1891.
[23] *ibid.*
[24] The *Cleckheaton and Spen Valley Guardian*, 8 May 1891.
[25] *Twenty-fourth Annual Report of the Local Government Board*, p. 49.
[26] The *Mirfield and Ravensthorpe Guardian*, 8 May 1891.
[27] The *Cleckheaton and Spen Valley Guardian*, 8 May 1891.
[28] St. Luke's National School log book, May & July 1891. West Yorkshire Archive Service (WYAS), Kirklees, RD53/6/4.
[29] *1892 Report of the Cleckheaton MOH*, WYAS (Wakefield) WRD 6/1/46.
[30] The *British Medical Journal*, 8 August, 1891, p.307.
[31] The *Dewsbury Reporter*, 9 May 1891.
[32] The *Dewsbury District News*, 9 May 1891.
[33] The *Dewsbury Reporter*, 9 May 1981.
[34] The *Cleckheaton and Spen Valley Guardian*, 15 May 1891.
[35] Cleckheaton Cemetery Burial Register, Kirklees Family History Library, Huddersfield: Microfiche.
[36] This information re Arthur Wood's birthplace came to light during a BBC Radio 3 weekend of light music, June 2011. A search through census returns confirmed my initial query.
[37] The *Spenborough Guardian and Heckmondwike Herald*, 23 January 1953.
[38] The *Cleckheaton Guardian*, 22 May 1891.
[39] The *Dewsbury Reporter*, 16 May 1891.
[40] *ibid.*
[41] *ibid,* 23 May 1891 and *Cleckheaton Guardian*, 22 May 1891.
[42] B. Wadsworth, *Edward Wadsworth: A Painter's Life,* (Michael Russell, 1989) p.2.
[43] *ibid*, p. 2.
[44] The *Dewsbury Reporter*, 23 May 1891.
[45] D. Linstrum, *West Yorkshire Architects and Architecture,* (Lund Humphries, 1978), p.355.
[46] *ibid,* p. 3.

Notes

[47] The *Cleckheaton and Spen Valley Guardian*, 5 June 1891.
[48] F. Peel, *Spen Valley Past and Present*, 1893 p. 374.
[49] J.M. Brooke, *The Story of a Church*, (St Luke's Vicar and Churchwardens, 1964) p. 28.
[50] The *Cleckheaton and Spen Valley Guardian*, 22 May 1891.
[51] I am grateful to Brenda Tatham for drawing my attention to the connection between Cleckheaton and Edward Wadsworth.
[52] Information related to household arrangements from 1891 census.
[53] J. Lewison (Ed), *The Genius of Industrial England*, (Arkwright Trust and Bradford Art Galleries and Museums, 1990). Back cover.
[54] I am grateful to Alex Hollweg, Edward Wadsworth's grandson, for this information.
[55] J. Greenwood, *The Graphic Work of Edward Wadsworth*, (The Wood Lea Press, 2002), p. 24.
[56] *ibid* and 12 June 1891.
[57] *Annual Report of the Huddersfield MOH*, 1892 (Huddersfield Library).
[58] MOH reports for Liversedge, Gomersal and Birkenshaw, for 1891: published 1892. (WYAS, Wakefield) refs: 6/1/178, 6/1/89, 6/1/22.
[59] *MOH report to Liversedge Local Board*, 1892 (WYAS ref 6/1/178).
[60] *MOH report to Gomersal Local Board*, 1892 (WYAS ref 6/1/89).
[61] *MOH report to Birkenshaw Local Board*, 1892 (WYAS ref 6/1/22).
[62] *MOH report to Cleckheaton Local Board*, 1892 (WYAS ref 6/1/46).
[63] *MOH Report to Bradford City Council*, 1892 (Bradford Reference Library).
[64] The *Cleckheaton and Spen Valley Guardian*, 5 June 1891.
[65] Gale, (1959), pp. 49-50.

Chapter Seven: When Panic Seized the Town

[1] *Pears Cyclopaedia*, (A. F. Pears Ltd., 1898; Pelham Books reprint, 1977), p.721.
[2] J.R. Smith, *The Speckled Monster*, (Essex Record Office, Chelmsford, 1987), p.15.
[3] C. Kotton, *A.D.A.M.'S Health Encyclopaedia*, (Boston, U.S.A: 2001)
[4] I. & J. Glynn, *The Life and Death of Smallpox*, (Profile Books, 2004) p. 73.
[5] P. Baughan, *North of Leeds*, (Roundhouse Books, London:1966), p. 175.
[6] T. Coleman, *The Railway Navvies*, (Penguin Books, London:1981), p. 224.
[7] S. Halliday, *The Great Filth*, (Sutton Publishing, 2007) p. 8.
[8] J.R. Smith, 1987, p. 15.
[9] S. Halliday, 2007, p. 8.
[10] I. & J. Glynn, *The Life and Death of Smallpox*, (Profile Books, 2004), p. 42.
[11] *Reports on Public Health and Medical Subjects*: No. 62, p. 6.
[12] I. Coulson & I. Dawson, *Medicine and Health Through Time* (John Murray, 1988) pp.115-117.
[13] H. Gordon, Letter to the *Daily Telegraph*, 16 October 2002.
[14] I. & J. Glynn, (2004), p. 39.
[15] B. Dolan, *Josiah Wedgwood*, (Harper Collins, 2004), p. 202.
[16] I. Coulson and I. Dawson, *Medicine and Health Through Time*, (1988) and M.

Henderson, 'Smallpox: The lethal choice we must face' (*The Times*, T2, 4 December, 2002).

[17] D. Crawford, *Deadly Companions,* (Oxford University Press, 2007), p.106.
[18] M. Henderson, (2002).
[19] The *Brighouse Echo*, 6 May 1892.
[20] The *Brighouse News*, 7 May 1892.
[21] *Report of the Medical Officer of Health to the Halifax Rural Sanitary Authority*, 31 December, 1892 (West Yorkshire Archive Service [Wakefield Headquarters] - *hereafter WYAS*-RD7/6/1/102).
[22] The *Brighouse Echo*, 13 May 1892.
[23] R. Mitchell, *Portrait of a Town,* (Brighouse Corporation, 1953) p. 183.
[24] The *Brighouse Echo*, 13 May 1892.
[25] The *Brighouse News*, 7 May 1892.
[26] Kelly's Directory, West Riding of Yorkshire, 1893, (Kelly and Co. London).
[27] *Report of MOH, Halifax Rural Sanitary Authority*, 31 Dec. 1892.
[28] The *Brighouse Echo*, 6 May 1892.
[29] *Report of MOH, Halifax Rural Sanitary Authority*, 31 Dec. 1892.
[30] Clifton St. John's School, Log Book,1892, (Clifton School).
[31] The *Brighouse Echo*, 6 May 1892.
[32] Clifton St. John's School, log book, 1892.
[33] *ibid.*
[34] *ibid.*
[35] The *Brighouse Echo*, 13 May 1892.
[36] *ibid.*
[37] *ibid.*
[38] *ibid.*
[39] *Report of MOH, Hipperholme Local Board*, 1893. (WYAS, RD7/6/1/123)
[40] *ibid*
[41] *Report of MOH, Southowram Urban Sanitary Authority*, 1892. (WYAS)
[42] The *Brighouse Echo*, 13 May 1892.
[43] *ibid,* 3 June 1892
[44] (i) Rastrick Infants' School log book. (WYAS [Calderdale] BG36).
(ii) St. Martin's Girls' School, Brighouse log book. (*ibid*. BG59).
(iii) Brookfoot School Log Book.(*ibid*. BG73).
(iv) Rastrick Common Boys' School (Rastrick High School).
(v) The *Brighouse News*, 28 May 1892.
(vi) *ibid*, 2 June 1892.
[45] The *Brighouse News*, 21 May 1892
[46] The *Brighouse Echo*, 20 May 1892.
[47] I am grateful to the late William Thrippleton for this information.
[48] The *Brighouse News*, 21 and 28 May 1892.
[49] (i) The *Brighouse Echo*, 3 June 1892.
(ii) The *Brighouse News*, 4 June 1892.
[50] The *Brighouse Echo*, 5 June 1892.
[51] The *Brighouse News*, 25 June 1892.
[52] The *Brighouse Echo*, 1 July 1892.
[53] *ibid*, 15 July 1892.
[54] The *Brighouse News*, 30 July 1892.

55. The *Brighouse Echo*, 17 June 1892.
56. I am grateful to Mrs Dorothy Holmes for this information that relates to her great-grandfather.
57. The *Brighouse News*, 23 July 1892.
58. *ibid*, 24 September 1892.
59. *ibid*, 25 November 1892.
60. *ibid*, 23 December 1892.
61. *ibid*, 17 June 1892.
62. Hipperholme Urban District Council Minutes, 1893 (WYAS [Calderdale] HIP 22).
63. *MOH Report, Hipperholme Local Board*, April, 1893 (WYAS,RD7/6/1/123).
64. *The Brighouse Echo*, 2 December 1892.
65. Hipperholme Local Board, minute book, 1874 – 1892 (WYAS [Calderdale] BRI490)
66. Lightcliffe St. Matthew's Parish Church magazine: February 1893.
67. *A Century of Bradford League Cricket, 1903-2003* - Brighouse CC supplement. (Bradford Cricket League, 2003).
68. *MOH Report, Hipperholme Local Board*, April 1893.
69. *MOH Report, Southowram Urban Sanitary Authority*, 1892 (WYAS).
70. *What was Happening in Brighouse 100 Years Ago*. (Brighouse Historical Society:1992).
71. The *Brighouse Echo*, 13 May 1892.
72. *ibid*, 12 August 1892.
73. *ibid*, 20 May 1892.
74. *Report of MOH, Borough of Brighouse,*1893. (WYAS, RD7/6/1/33).
75. The *Brighouse Echo*, 20 May 1892.
76. (i) *ibid*, 13 May 1892.
    (ii) Rastrick Common Boys' School Logbook (Rastrick High School).
77. The *Brighouse Echo*, 13 May 1892.
78. *ibid*, 20 May 1892.
79. I am grateful to Miss Isobel Sutcliffe for this information.
80. Rastrick Infants' School logbook.
81. Royal Society for the Protection of Birds, *Birds,* magazine. Autumn, 2011.
82. J. R. Smith,1987, p. 93 & E. A. Underwood et al, *Edward Jenner: The Man and his Work,* (The Jenner Trust, 1949)
83. I. & J. Glynn, (2004), p43-46; S. Halliday, (2007), pp. 9-10.
84. M. Dobson, *Disease*, (Quercus, 2007), p. 134.
85. The *Brighouse Echo*, 3 June 1892.
86. Rastrick Infants' School logbook .
87. R. Mitchell, *Birth and Death of a Borough*, (The Ridings Publishing Co. Driffield: 1976), p. 83.
88. *MOH Report, Brighouse Local Board*, 1892. (WYAS, RD7/6/1/33).
89. *ibid*.
90. www.mayoclinic.com.
91. R. Mitchell, *Portrait of a Town, (*Brighouse Corporation: 1953*)*, p. 183.
92. The *Brighouse Echo*, 13 May 1892.
93. *ibid,*
94. *ibid*, 24 June 1892.

95 *ibid*, 20 May 1892.
96 *ibid*, 27 May 1892.
97 The *Brighouse News*, 28 May 1892.
98 The *Brighouse Echo*, 3 June 1892.
99 The *Brighouse News*, 4 June 1892.
100 The *Brighouse Echo*, 17 June 1892.
101 *ibid,* 24 June 1892.
102 The *Brighouse Echo*,15 July 1892.
103 Letter from Brighouse Joint Hospital Board, 4 April, 1894. (WYAS, RD7/6/1/35).
104 *ibid*.
105 Letter from Local Government Board to Brighouse Joint Hospital Board, 26 July 1894, (WYAS, RD7/6/1/35).
Report of Brighouse Corporation Conference, 5 February, 1895.
106 C. Helme, 'Centenary of Queen Victoria's Death' (*Brighouse Echo*, 22 January 2001).
107 County Borough of Halifax, *Report on the Epidemic of Smallpox in the years, 1892-3.*
J. B. Eagles, *Smallpox in the Holme Valley, 1892-39* (retained at the Jenner Museum, Berkeley**).**
108 The *Daily Telegraph*, 11 December 1979.
109 K. McCarthy, 'The End of Smallpox?', *The Bulletin of the Liverpool Medical History Society*, no. 19, 2007-08, p.11-16.

Chapter Eight: A Baffling Outbreak

1 L.A. Sawchuk, in *Plagues and Epidemics,* D.A. Herring and A.C. Swedland, (Eds), (A. & C. Black, 2010), p. 95.
2 St. Stephen's School Log Book, (School Archives).
3 Woodroyd Boys' School Log Book (West Yorkshire Archive Service, Bradford. Ref: 48D000)
4 A. Hardy, *The Epidemic Streets*, (Clarendon Press,p.81) and R. Woods and N. Shelton, *An Atlas of Victorian Mortality,* (Liverpool University Press, 1997), p. 57.
5 M. Greenwood, *Epidemics and Crowd Diseases,* (Williams & Norgate, 1935), p. 197.
6 Hardy, (1993), p. 82.
7 A.H. Gale, *Epidemic Disease,* (Pelican, 1959), p. 93.
8 F.B. Smith, *The People's Health,1830-1910,* (Weidenfeld & Nicolson, 1990), p.149.
9 Hardy, (1993), p. 86.
10 A.S. Wohl, *Endangered Lives,* (Methuen, 1983), p. 129.
11 Hardy, (1993), p. 102.
12 *ibid*, pp.82-3.
13 Wohl, (1983), p. 130.
14 Smith, (1990), p.151.
15 Hardy, (1993), p. 109.
16 *ibid,* p. 100.

[17] *ibid,* p. 150.
[18] Hardy, (1993), p. 87.
[19] A. Newsholme, *The Origin and Spread of Pandemic Diphtheria,* (Swan Sounenschein, 1898), pp. 40-1.
[20] The *Bradford Weekly Telegraph,* 1 & 8 October 1904.
[21] B. Thompson, 'Infant mortality in nineteenth-century Bradford', p.139 in R. Woods, and J. Woodward, (Eds), *Urban Disease and Mortality in Nineteenth Century England,* (Batsford, 1984).
[22] Evans, (1904), pp.42-3.
[23] W. A. Evans, *MOH Report on the Prevalence of Diphtheria in Bradford,* (1904).
[24] *ibid.*
[25] Evans, (1904), p. 45.
[26] I am grateful to William Baines for much of this information.
[27] 1891 Census, Bowling St. Stephen's Parish: Tennant Street.
[28] W. Cudworth, *Histories of Bolton and Bowling,* pp. 244-46.
[29] *ibid.*
[30] *ibid.*
[31] Greenwood, (1935), pp. 198-99.
[32] Hardy, (1993), p. 88.
[33] E.W. Goodhall et al, *Scarlet Fever, Diphtheria and Enteric Fever,1895-1914* quoted by Hardy, 1993, p. 89.
[34] Evans, (1904), p. 49.
[35] W. Angus, *MOH Report on the health and sanitary administration of the City for the year 1918,* (City of Leeds)

Chapter Nine: An Unwelcome Present from Scarborough

[1] The *Huddersfield Weekly Examiner,* 5 November 1932.
[2] A.H. Gale, *Epidemic Diseases,* (Pelican, 1959) cites an outbreak in Bournemouth and Poole, when there were 518 typhoid cases in 1936, as an example of a milk-borne outbreak.
[3] G. Gill et al, *Public Health and Public Paranoia: the 1888 typhoid outbreak in Wallasey.* The Local Historian, February, 2005, p. 21.
[4] F.B. Smith, *The People's Health,* (Weidenfield & Nicolson, 1990), p. 244.
[5] D.H. Crawford, *Deadly Companions* (Oxford University Press, 2007), p. 156.
[6] A.S. Wohl, *Endangered Lives,* (Methuen, 1983), p. 127.
[7] S. Halliday, *The Great Filth,* (Sutton Publishing, 2007), pp. 71-72.
[8] *ibid.*
[9] Wohl, (1983), p. 127.
[10] Smith, (1990), p. 245.
[11] Halliday, (2007), pp. 69-71.
[12] Wohl, (1983), p. 128.
[13] I am grateful to William and Susan Cooper for this information relating to the property's name.
[14] I am grateful to John Springer for initially drawing my attention to this information, that is confirmed in *Plain Country Friends: Short Walks from High Flatts,* a short walks leaflet produced by Denby Dale Parish Council,

Kirklees Council and 'Discover East Peak'.
[15] I am grateful to Arthur Pritchard and John Springer for this information.
[16] I am grateful to the family of Kate Robson, especially her grandson James Anderson, for so readily allowing me to include this information, and for being so helpful with my research.
[17] D. Bower, and J. Knight, *Plain Country Friends*, (Wooldale Meeting of the Religious Society of Friends, 1987), pp. 107,109,145 & *A Brief History of High Flatts Meeting House*, (leaflet at Meeting House).
[18] The *Holmfirth Express*, 22 October 1932.
[19] *ibid*.
[20] St. John the Evangelist Church, Denby, burial records, microfiche ref 2237, Huddersfield Local History Library.
[21] St. Nicholas's Church, Cumberworth, burial records, Huddersfield Local History Library, microfiche 2245, sheet 11452 and St. John's Church, Denby.
[22] The Penistone electoral roll, 1932. Township of Denby, Polling District AF: nos. 279 & 286 WYAS (Wakefield).
[23] The *Huddersfield Weekly Examiner*, 12 November 1932.
[24] *ibid* and the *Huddersfield Weekly Examiner*.
[25] The *Huddersfield Weekly Examiner*, 29 October 1932.
[26] The *Huddersfield Weekly Examiner*, 22 October 1932.
[27] C Heath, *Denby and District*, Wharncliffe Books, (2004). p. 217.
[28] The *Huddersfield Examiner*, 3 November 1932.
[29] *ibid*, 3 and 19 November 1932.
[31] The *Huddersfield Weekly Examiner*, 22 October.
[32] The *Barnsley Chronicle*, 29 October 1932.
[33] The *Huddersfield Weekly Examiner*, 22 October & 19 November.
[34] *ibid*, 22 October.
[35] Information from the Holy Trinity Church website, 2012.
[36] *Forty-fourth Annual Report of the County Medical Officer*, County Hall Wakefield, 1932, p.15, West Yorkshire Archive Service (WYAS) WRD7/1/1/45.
[37] The *Holmfirth Express*, 22 October 1932.
[38] The information relating to the dates that mills were established was gleaned from a local information board at Denby Dale Railway Station and bus interchange.
[39] The *Huddersfield Weekly Examiner*, 22 October 1932.
[40] *ibid*.
[41] The *Barnsley Chronicle*, 29 October 1932.
[42] The *Huddersfield Examiner*, 20 October 1932.
[43] The *British Medical Journal*, 28 January 1933.
[44] The *Holmfirth Express*, 22 October 1932.
[45] *ibid*, 29 October.
[46] *ibid*.
[47] *ibid*, 5 November.
[48] Denby Dale District Council School Log Book, 1921-45 WYAS, (Kirklees), CW/E/DD/6 & Victoria Hall Infants' School Log Book, RD/53/6/7
[49] Denby Dale District Council School Log Book, 1921-45.
[50] The *Holmfirth Express*, 5 November 1932.
[51] *ibid*, 29 October.

Notes

52 *ibid*, 5 November.
53 The *Huddersfield Examiner*, 29 October 1932.
54 The *Barnsley Chronicle*, 29 October 1932.
55 I am grateful to the descendants of Ernest Lockwood, George Parker and Doreen Wood for their help in compiling this family tree and for allowing me to publish it.
56 Denby and Cumberworth Council Minutes, 22 December, 1932, p. 295, WYAS, (Kirklees), WRD 7/6/2/30.
57 The *Barnsley Chronicle*, 29 October 1932.
58 *Report on an Outbreak of Enteric Fever in the Malton Urban District*, (Reports on Public Health and Medical Subjects, no. 69), 1933.
59 The *Holmfirth Express*, 5 November 1932.
60 *ibid*.
61 St. Nicholas's Church, Cumberworth, burial records.
62 The *Holmfirth Express*, 5 November 1932.
63 I am extremely grateful to Mrs. Mary Lockwood for this information and the help given by her son Michael in making this possible.
64 The *Huddersfield Weekly Examiner*, 5 November 1932.
65 *Forty-fourth Annual Report of the County Medical Officer*, (1932).
66 The *Huddersfield Examiner*, 19 October 1932.
67 I am grateful to Nev Leah for his work on this image.
68 I am grateful to William Cooper for this information.
69 The *Huddersfield Weekly Examiner*, 5 November.
70 *Forty-fourth Annual Report of the County Medical Office*, (1932).
71 T. Smith, *Denby Dale School: 1874-1974*, (Parent-Teacher Association), p. 14.
72 *Report of the Huddersfield MOH*, 1933, p. 77.
73 The *Medical Officer*, Vol. 48, 19 November 1932, p. 214.
74 Eyler, John M., *Sir Arthur Newsholme and State Medicine, 1885-1935*, (Cambridge University Press, 1997), pp. 119-20.
75 The *Huddersfield Weekly Examiner*, 5 & 19 November.
76 *ibid*, 19 November.
77 The *Barnsley Chronicle*, 29 October 1932.
78 Denby and Cumberworth Council Minutes, p. 284.
79 The *Holmfirth Express*, 19 November 1932.
80 *British Medical Journal*, 3 December 1932, p. 1038.
81 Denby and Cumberworth Council Minutes, 1 December 1932, p. 282.
82 *ibid*, 22 December, 1932, p. 294.
83 *ibid*, 12 January, 1933, p. 302.
84 *ibid*, 22 December, 1932, p. 294, & 9 March, 1933, p. 317.
85 *ibid*.
86 *ibid*, 18 August, 1932, p. 260.
87 WRD/6/1/57, Files 3126 & 3320.
88 The *Huddersfield Examiner*, 3 December 1932, & St. Nicholas's Church burial records.
89 The *Huddersfield Examiner*, 19 October 1932.
90 I am grateful to Ron Jackson for this information.
91 Denby and Cumberworth Council Minutes, 1932, p. 220.
92 T. W. Woodhead, *A History of Huddersfield Water Supplies*, (Tolson Memorial

Museum Publications, 1939), p. 99.
[93] I am grateful to Lynn Gill, archivist at Yorkshire Water, for this information.
[94] J. Addy (ed), *A History of Denby Dale Urban District*, (Denby Dale UDC, 1973), p. 35.

Index

Ainley, Dr. D. 54, 55, 57, 63, 64, 65, 67, 68, 87, 88
Akroyd, Edward 4
Akroyd, J. 49
Allbutt, C. 6
Angus, Dr. W. 122
Anning, S. T. 38
Arkwright, R. 3
Armstrong, M. 36, 37
Armytage Arms, Clifton 101
Ayrey, R. 36

Bailey, I. 48
Bailiff Bridge 141
Baines, E. 35
Bairstow, H. 101
Baker, Dr. R. 26-30, 32, 33, 36, 37, 41, 43
Baker, J. 103
Baldwin, E. 101
Ballard, Dr. 65
Barnard, S. 29, 41
Barnsley Chronicle 130
Barrett Browning, E. 11
Barwick Green 76
Batley 70, 73
Beevers, A. 136
Beevers, J. 93
Bell, R. 55, 57, 65, 66
Belper 3
Beresford, M. D. 10, 24, 30
Berkeley 102-103
Bickerdyke, J. 93, 109
Birkenshaw 71, 72, 75, 81, 82
Birmingham 4
Birmingham Medical School 109
Birstall 70
Birthwhistle, Dr. R. 34
Blackburn 4
Blackshaw Head 49
Bleasdell, Dr. J. T. 128, 130, 136, 138, 142
Bond, Dr. F. F. 100, 101, 104
Bordeaux 12
Bottomley, I. 93, 109
Bottomley, Taylor 93

Bottomley, Thomas 106
Bournville 4
Bowling Brick Works 117
Bradford 1, 2, 4, 6, 41, 43, 100, 108 111, 113, 114, 122
  infant mortality 114
  Woodroyd Brick Works 116
  Woodroyd School 111, 116
  Cross Lane School 116
  Ryan Street School 116
  St. Joseph's School 116
  St. Stephen's School 116, 117
Bransgrove, F. 133
Briggs, A. 43
Briggs, Samuel and family 83, 87, 88, 90, 108
Brighouse, Bethel Street 96
  Bradford Road 97
  Clifton Common 90, 101
  Commercial Street 94-95
  Co-operative 92
  Daisy Croft 83, 87, 91, 92, 94, 109
  'ghost town' 83, 92
  Haigh Street 95
  King Street 91, 93
  Lane Head 92
  Park Street 95, 99
  Police Street 91, 93, 94, 109
  Vaccination Committee 101
Brighouse Echo 86, 87, 89, 93, 94, 95, 96, 101, 104, 106, 109
Brighouse News 88, 94, 96, 97, 107
Brighton 2, 68, 140
Bristol 125
British Medical Journal 54, 55, 56, 57, 65
Britton, Dr. T. 64, 65
brochitis 72, 80, 82
Brockington, F. 31
Bronte, E. 11
Brook, E. 127-128
Brookfoot 91, 92
Brooks family 17
Broomfield House 78
Broomfield Mills 77, 78
Brown, J. F. 106

Brown, J.L. 31, 32
Budd, W. 125
Burke, Mrs. 38
Burnett, J. 2, 5, 9
Burnley, C. & J. 73
Butler, Miss 134

Cadbury, G.& R. 4
Calder Valley 47
Calverley 139
Cameron, Dr. J.S. 18-19
Campbell, Dr. 80
Carter, Dr. 87
cellar dwellings 45
Chadwick, E. 4, 5, 27, 41
Chapel-le-Dale 83
Charteris, Dr. 97
Chesterfield, Earl of 124
chicken pox 62
Child, H. 83, 88
Child, Rev. J. 90
cholera 1, 8, 10, 22-43, 108
cholera riots 36, 41-3
cholera, cures and medicines 32-6
cholera, Leeds Epidemic 22-43
cholera, symptoms 23
Churchill, J.F. 11
Clayton West U.D.C. 136
Clayton, J. 97
Cleckheaton 72, 73, 74, 75, 76, 78, 81, 82
   Cemetery 76, 78
   Brooke Street School 77
   Central Methodist Church 77
   Providence Place Church 78
   St. Luke's School 74
   Town Hall 77
   well-known families 78
   Westgate Cong. Church 78,
Cleckheaton and Spen Valley Guardian 73, 75, 80, 82
Clifton 76, 83, 85-8, 90, 92, 94, 95, 98, 100, 105, 109
   hospital 83, 87-8
   school 89-91, 109
   Collier Row 91
   Grave Lane 90
   Kiln Fold 91, 93, 95, 110

   Savile Lane 83, 87-91, 91, 93, 100, 101, 109
   Thornhills Lane 90, 106, 108
   Vine House Farm 83
   Woodhead Lane 101
Colden Valley 49
Coley 98
consumption (see tuberculosis)
Cook, D. 137
Cooper family 16
Copley 4
Cowan, R. 5
cowpox 85-6, 101-2
Craven, B. 77
Crawford, J.H. 13
Creese, W. 4
Creighton, C. 12, 55
Crewe 3
Cromford, 3
Crossland, J. 127
Crossley, F. 4
Cudworth, W. 117

Dale, D. 3
Dargue, J. and M. 76
Dawson, Dr. R. 98
Day, A. 15
death, age of, rate 3, 12, 14, 15, 16, 18, 20, 33, 42, 45, 46, 47, 51, 52
Delaine, Mr. 89
Denby Dale 1,15
   Co-operative Terrace 128, 134
   Council School 130
   Brownhill's Mill 131
   Hartcliffe View 133
   Hinchliffe's (Hartcliffe) Mill 130, 137
   Kenyon's Mill 130
   Park View 133
   Polygon Terrace 144
   Prospect Hotel 131
   Rockwood Hall 144
   School Terrace 137
   Smithroyd 136
   St. Nicholas's Church 133, 136
   U.D.C. 136, 145, 146
   White Hart Hotel 131
Denby and Cumberworth U.D.C 123,

128, 130, 136, 140
Denby Dale and Cumberworth
   Station 142
Denham, Mr. 94
Dewsbury 70, 72, 73, 75
Dewsbury Reporter 73, 75
Dewsnap, E. R. 9
Dicey and Co. 34
Dickens, C. 8, 45
Dickinson, J. 100
Dickinson, J. 100,
diphtheria 1, 10, 11, 111-22
   cures 121
   symptoms 112
Dock, J. 31
Dolan, Dr. 65
Doncaster 23, 37, 67
Driffield 72
Dufton, J. 25
Durey, M. 22, 38

Easton, Rev. E.W. 78
Eccleshill 114
Edwards, Dr. B. 98
Elland 98
Ellis, F. 80
Ematt, T. 96
Emley U.D.C. 136
Engels, F. 6, 35
English sweat 70
Evans, Dr. B. A. 111, 116, 119
Exley Gate 144

Fallowfield 56,
Farr, W. 5
Farrand, H. 89, 90, 95
Fawcett, R. 31
Felton, Mr. 35
Figures, G. 46
Finsbury 6
Fisher, C. 128
Forsyth, Dr. R. A. 81

Gale, A. H. 82
Gardner family 16
Gaskell. E. 8
Gelder family 97
Gill, G. 123

Gill, G. & Burrell, A. S. 42
Gledhill, G. 73
Gledhill, W. and P. 61
Gledhill. E. 59, 60
Glossop, C. 136
Gomersal 71, 72, 75, 81, 82
Goole 22
Goring, J. 90
Gouldie, E. 4
Goux closets 61, 62
Grace, H. 125
grave robbing 36-38
Grave, J. 24
Greasbrough 139
Great Horton 115
Great Northern Railway 60
'Green Hollows' 126, 137
Greenwood, J. 79
Greenwood, T. 48
Greg, Samuel 3
Gregory, Dr. G. 10

Hackney 6
Hague, W. 12
Halifax 2, 4, 8, 10, 47, 53-69, 113
   Ashfield Terrace 59
   Aspinall Street 58
   Bull Green 59
   Coton Street 59
   Craven Terrace 58, 59
   Fever Hospital 87, 89, 90, 109
   Gerrard Street 58
   Gibbet Street 59
   Hopwood Lane 56, 58, 59, 61
   National School 61
   Pellon Lane Infants' School 61
   Queens Rd. Infants, School 61, 62
   Queen's Road 59
   Roils Head 61
   Rural Sanitary Authority 87, 88,
   101, 105
   St. Augustine's School 61
   St. Paul's Station 59
   Vickerman Street 58
Halifax Courier 58, 61, 63
Halifax Guardian 53, 58, 59, 61, 64,
   65
Hamburg 23

hand loom weavers 48-9
Handel, D. 117-19
Hardy, A. 11, 45
Harrison, Rev. A. 98
Harrogate 31
Hartshead, parish of 90
Haworth 5, 139
Hebden Bridge 47, 49
Heckmondwike 70, 73, 74, 75, 76, 82
   Cemetery 75, 76
   Boothroyd Lane School 75
   George Street 76
   Upper Ind. Chapel 73
   Westgate 76
Heptonstall 47
Heptonstall Slack 44-52
Hesketh, William 4
Hey, W. 23, 30
Hicks, C. 144
High Flatts 123, 126
Highfield House 78
Hill, Rev. G. 104
Hinchliffe, J. 130, 136, 144, 146
Hipperholme 91, 97, 98, 99
Hipperholme Infants' School 13
Hirst, F. and E. 128
Holbeck 15, 24, 26, 34
Holdsworth, J. 77
Hole, J. 3, 6
Hollins Hey Hospital 98
Holt, B. and M. 48
Honigsbaum, M. 71
Horn, F. 145
Horsfield, W. 57, 64. 65, 67, 68
hospitals 4, 13, 26, 31, 32, 34, 35, 36, 39, 40, 41, 83, 87-88, 127, 128,
housing 1, 4, 6, 8, 9, 10,15,16, 19, 20,24, 25, 27, 41, 42, 49, 51
housing, back to back 9, 10, 19, 73
Hove Edge 96, 105
Howard, R. 44, 45, 47, 48, 49, 50, 51
Howarth, J. 48
Hoyle, Mr. 59
Huddersfield 2, 4, 6, 80, 125, 126, 128, 133, 138, 139, 146
Huddersfield (Mill Hill) Hospital 128, 130, 133

Huddersfield Daily Examiner 128, 130, 137, 141, 144
Huddersfield Weekly Examiner 128, 138
Hughes, T 24, 48
Hull 22, 23, 38, 39, 41, 72
Humber Estuary 22
Hunslet 23, 24, 26
Hutchins, J. 38

Idle 114
Ilkley 31
Ilkley, Godby's School 78
influenza 20, 70-1, 74-5, 80-2
   symptoms 71
Ireland 45

Jackson, R. 145
Jacques, M.and A. 144
Jenner, E.
Johnson, S. 35

Kay, J. 31, 32
Keats, J. 11
Keenan, T. and E. 46
Kell, Dr. J. B. 22
Kendle, J. 24
Kennally, H. 45
King, Rev. T. 88
Kirkburton Hospital 128, 137
Knostrop 24
Knowling, G. 14
Koch, R. 5, 8, 11

Lampard, E. 5
Lancet 30, 34, 137
Lane, J. 99
Laundon, A. and R. 127-28
Law, J. 80
Lawson Road 94
Leamington Spa 27
Leeds 2, 3, 4, 5, 6, 7, 8, 9, 10, 12, 14, 24-43, 44, 45, 46, 52, 139
   Anatomy School 34
   Armley 36-37
   Back York Street 45
   Blue Bell Fold 24, 29, 39, 41, 42
   Board of Health 23, 24, 26, 27, 40,

Index

41, 42, 43
Boot and Shoe Yard 3, 24, 25, 27, 31, 32, 39, 40, 41
Bridge 15
Briggate 29, 34, 38
Brighton Court 45
Bull and Mouth, Hotel 38
Burmantofts 32
cellar dwellings 28, 45, 46
Duke Street 15
East Ardsley 38
East Ward 45
Ebenezer St. 16
Fleece Lane 28
Foundry Street 45
Goulden's Buildings 45
House of Correction 40, 41
House of Recovery 6, 23, 29
Hunslet Lane 14, 15
Improvement Act 42
Kirkgate 15, 16, 18, 24, 29, 35, 45
Lower Cross St. 45
Mabgate 15
Marsh Lane 14, 15, 16, 20, 34
Oulton 38
Parish Church 14, 17, 31, 45, 46
Quarry Hill 15, 16, 18, 24, 28
Richmond Road 28
Riley's Yard 6
Royal Oak Yard 24
Saxton Lane 40
School of Medicine 34
St. Peters Square 39
The Bank 15, 16, 18, 23, 24, 31, 32, 45, 49
Timble Beck 42
Vicar Lane 39
Water Lane 15
yards and folds 24, 25, 28, 31, 32, 42
York Road 15, 18
York Street 24, 25, 28
Off Street 15
Leeds Intelligencer 22, 23, 34, 35, 38, 39, 42
Leeds Mercury 6, 14, 23, 25, 30, 35
Leeds Road Hospital 114

Leeson, Mrs. M. 39, 40
Leicester 4
Lever, W. H. 4
Lewis, P. W. 55, 79
Lightcliffe 12
Lille 12
Lister, J. 5
Little Horton 115
Liverpool 2, 3, 5, 22, 45, 106
Liversedge 71, 72, 73, 81, 82, 89
Local Government Boards 12, 18, 19
Lockwood, A. and M. 134
Lockwood, E. 133
Lockwood, M. 136-137
Londesborough, Earl of 124
London 1, 2, 4, 6, 8, 22, 113
Lower Denby 144
Luddenden 57, 65
Lumb Mills 49
Lydgate, Lightcliffe 97, 98, 110

Magee, Archbishop 71
Mallon, M. 123-124
Malton 72, 131, 136, 141, 142
Manchester 2, 4, 5, 8, 31, 38
Manningham 115, 119
Market Weighton 22
Mayhall, J 38
measles 10, 11, 12-21, 62, 83, 114
    symptoms 13
Medical Officer Journal 140
Meltham Hospital 127, 128, 133, 137
Metcalf, J. 85
Micklethwaite, R. 18
Middlesborough 4
Midgeley 48
Midland Railway 54, 84
Miller Hill Chapel 136
Monck, W.S. 46
Montagu Wortley, Lady M. 103
Morley, Mr. 34, 39
Morrison, Dr. R. 74, 82
Mosley, G.S. 130, 136
Munchcliffe Dyke (Beck) 137-38
Murphy, S. 121
Mytholmroyd 48

Napoleon. 45

175

Nelmes, S. 103
New Lanark 3
New York 67
Newbold, Mrs. 94
Newcastle 30
Newsholme, A. 68, 140
Newton, George 6
Niblett, L. 96
Noble, T. and R. 133
North Bierley Hospital 114
Norwich 2
Norwood Green 98

Oakenshaw 77
Oddy, M. 34, 37
Ogden, W. and J. 15
Oldfield, G. 89
Owen, R. 3

Paisley 38
Paley, R. 117
Parker, E. 133
Parker, G. 134
Parker, J. 109
Parker, P. and M. 134
Parson, Dr. F. 74
Pasteur, L. 5
Payne, T. 97
Peace, L. S. 128
Pears Cyclopaedia 13, 83
Penistone 126
Penistone Hospital 128, 134, 136, 146
Phipps, J. 103
Pilling, W. 106
Pindar, P.K.G. 140
Plath, S. 47
pneumonia 10, 11, 71, 72, 80, 82
population growth 1, 3
Port Sunlight 4
Potts, Dr. T.N.V. 137
power looms 48
Power, Sir W. 119
Preston 4, 8
Priest, L. and F. 137
Priestley, Mr. 98
Pringle, Sir J. 29
Prowazeki S, von 45

Quaker Bottom 123, 126, 127, 137, 139, 146
Queen Victoria 2, 4, 5, 6

Ramsden, C. 101
Ramsden, N. 14
Ramsden, R. 90, 105
Ranger, W. 8, 10
Rape, M. 45
Rastrick 83, 87, 90, 93, 94, 96, 98, 105, 106, 108, 109
   Church Infants' School 93
   Common School 92
   Grammar School 92
   Methodist Church 104
   Brick and Tile Terrace 96
   Firth Street 90, 100, 109
Redman, A. and E. 95, 110
Rickets, H.T. 45
Ripley, G and E. 117
Ripley's Dye Works 117
River Aire 6, 16, 22, 24, 41
Roberts, J. 94
Roberts, Miss 96
Robson, G. B. 126
Robson, K. 125-7, 137
Robson, W. T. 126
Royal Sanitary commission 37
Rusby Wood 136, 140, 142
Ruskin, J. 7, 11
Russia 70, 71, 75, 82
Russian influenza 70, 71, 75

Salford 4
'salt pie' houses 19
Salt, T. 4
sanitation 3, 4, 5, 6, 8, 10, 25, 42, 45, 121
Sawchuk, L. 111
Scarborough 123, 125, 126, 137, 138, 140, 146
scarlet fever 1, 10, 11, 83, 114, 120
   symptoms 53
Scholes 77
Scott, F. 95
Scott, H. H. 66, 67
Selby 22, 23, 24, 27
Semple, Dr. R. 112

sewers/sewerage 7, 8, 27, 28, 29, 30, 49-51, 123, 137, 145
Shann, A. 18
Sharpe, F. 35
Shaw, T. 99
Sheffield 41, 71, 72
Shepley, M. 130
Shepley, S. 130, 131, 133, 139, 144
Shires, Dr. J. 81
Shutt, E.and J. 31
Simmonds J. 24
Simon, J. 4, 34
Skelmanthorpe U.D.C. 136
Slack, J. and G. 80
Slade School of Art 79
smallpox 1, 10, 11, 12, 13, 16, 18, 62, 63
    effects of 85
    first cases in Brighouse 83, 86-7, 109
    history of 84-5
    innoculation 103
    symptoms 102
    vaccination 85-6, 101-2
Smith, B. 95
Smith, D.V. 28, 30, 35, 40
Smith, J. R. 6
Smith, R. 54
Smith, S. 41
Smith, Samuel 30
Smith, T, 36, 37, 38
Smith, T. S. 6, 29, 35
Snow,J. 28-29
Southowram 83, 92, 96, 98, 105
Spanish influenza 71
Spen Valley 70-7, 80, 81, 82
Spenborough U.D.C. 72, 140
Sproat,W. 22
Square Wood Reservoir 123, 127, 130, 136, 137, 139, 140, 142
St. Matthew's, Lightcliffe 98
St. Paul's Church, Kings Cross 59
St. Petersburg 71
Staincliffe 73
Stalin, J. 85
Steadman, Rev. R.P. 100
Steele, Dr. H. O. 75, 81
Stevenson, Robert Louis 10

Stewart, Dr. 73
Stoney Royd Isolation Hospital 63, 87, 90, 96, 97, 98, 101, 105, 106, 107, 109
Strutt. J. 3
Sturges, J. 117
Styal 3
Sunderland 22
Sutcliffe, I. 102
Sutton 126
Swann, Dr. 73
Swindon 2
Sykes, J. 97, 98
Sykes, J.H. 97

Tait, A. 54
Taylor, J. 90, 92, 93, 100, 109
Taylor, M 31
Teale, Mr. 34
Thackrah, C.T. 34, 36, 43
'The Archers' 76
Thomas.W. 40
Thornhill Briggs 95, 97
Thrippleton, B. 93, 94, 109
Tilling, R.H. 126
Tilling, T. 126
Tingle, E. 136
Tomlinson, J. 89-90
Tompkins, B. 142
Travis, Mr. 59
Tripe, Dr. 6
tuberculosis 10, 11, 34, 38, 95, 96, 114
Turkington & Co. 34
Turner, H. J. 101
typhoid 1, 10, 11, 44-52, 63, 123-47
    symptoms 65
typhus 1, 10, 11, 44-52, 104, 108, 124
    symptoms 44, 51-2

Underwood, E.A. 24, 29, 31
Urquhart, J. 31, 32

Vermont 67
Vorticist Movement 79

Waddington, L. 108

Wadsworth, B. 77
Wadsworth, Edward 55, 78-9
Wadsworth, Elymas 77-8
Wadsworth, H. 78
Wainwright, F. 136
Wakefield 2, 23, 40, 41, 88
Walton, E. 96
Walton, W. 117
Warley Hospital 98
Warley, 57, 63, 66
Warwick, E. 46
Water supply 7, 8, 9, 25, 26, 29, 44, 49, 50, 52
Watling, J. 97
Watson, T. 56
weavers 48-49
Wedgwood, J. 85-86
West Bowling 111, 114, 116, 117, 119, 121
West Bowling occupations 117
West, Rev. C. A. 145
Whindle, W. 32
Whitehall Inn, Hipperholme 97
Whitelegge, Dr. B.A. 14, 18, 20
Whiteley, J.W. 31
whooping cough 10, 11, 12, 13, 14, 18, 114
Wilson, W. 31, 34
Wohl, A. S. 113, 123, 124
Wood, A. H. 76
Wood, C. 134
Wood, D. 134
Wood, J. 76
Wood, Rev. O. A. 134
Wood, W.H. 61
workhouse 16, 36

York 2, 23
Yorkshire Gazette, 30

List of Subscribers

Thank you to the following people and organisations that have supported this publication:

Names		**Location**
Abernethy,	Lesley	Kelso
Armitage,	Mavis	Soyland
Asher,	Sue and Howard	Huddersfield
Baines,	William	Bradford
Beadle,	Ray and Sheena	Scarborough
Bennett,	Gemma and Paul	Copley
Bescoby,	Barbara	Sowerby Bridge
Bickerdike,	Maggie and Ivan	Lightcliffe
Brahney,	Margaret	Golcar
Brill,	Douglas	Northowram
Brooke,	Michael	Hipperholme
Brooke,	Simon and Caroline	Nafferton
Brough,	Ann	Liversedge
Cameron,	Iain	Halifax
Chambers,	Melanie and Steven	Halifax
Connolly,	Eileen	Northowram
Cook,	David	High Flatts
Costello,	Katie and Matthew	Hipperholme
Crabtree,	Barbara and Philip	Dalton, Huddersfield
Croft,	Linda	Todmorden
Davies,	Valerie	Marsh
Depelle,	Jacqueline G.	Yorkshire
Downing,	Betty	Addingham
Dunne,	Maureen	Keighley
Ellis,	Trevor and Colleen	Marsh
Emmerson,	Sally	Bradford
Farmer,	Christine	Bramhope
Fewster,	Malcolm and Trees	Gomersal
Ford,	Pauline	Shipley
Grassam,	Richard and Hannah	Scarborough
Greenwood,	Alan and Angela	Lightcliffe
Griffiths,	David	Huddersfield
Halifax Antiquarian Society		Halifax
Halmshaw,	John and Sylvia	Northallerton
Hargreaves,	Susan and John	Halifax
Harrison,	David and Jenny	Norwood Green
Helme,	Chris and Barbara	Lightcliffe
Hickin,	Philip and Lynne	Hipperholme
Holland,	Michael	Southend-on-Sea
Hollweg,	Alexander	Nettlecombe, Somerset

Holmes,	Dorothy	Lower Wyke
Horne,	Bob and Claire	Lightcliffe
Howard,	Elizabeth	Brighouse
Howard,	Ralph	Lightcliffe
Howes,	Stephen and Susan	Holmfirth
Illand,	David	Brighouse
Jackson,	Ronald and Margaret	Thornton-in-Craven
King,	Janis and Barry	Huddersfield
Kirker,	Anne	Rishworth
Kneeshaw,	Margaret	Liversedge
Knowles,	Philip and Lynn	Hipperholme
Lawton,	Kelvin and Janet	Clifton
Leach,	John and Jenny	Rastrick
Leah,	Liz and Nev	Lightcliffe
Lightcliffe Local History Society		Lightcliffe
Liverpool School of Tropical Medicine		Liverpool
Lockwood,	Mary	Skelmanthorpe
Lockwood,	Michael and Beryl	Shepley
Lodge,	Lynda and Martin	Rastrick
Luxton,	John and Jane	Leeds
Metcalfe,	David	Leeds
Mitchell,	Jill and Grayham	Lightcliffe
Natton,	Barry and Carole	Birkenhead
Naylor,	Frank and Jean	Liversedge
Normanton,	Katie	Leeds
Nortcliffe,	David and Margaret	Hipperholme
Northowram Historical Society		Northowram
Park,	Trevor	Rastrick
Parker,	Marjorie	Denby Dale
Petford,	Alan	Hipperholme
Polotnianka,	Mike and Jane	Huddersfield
Rhodes,	Penny	Otley
Rooke,	Derrick	Mirfield
Sharp,	Michael and Margaret	Brighouse
Sheead,	Stanley	Skelmanthorpe
Smith,	David and Linda	Lightcliffe
Stephenson,	Michael and Barbara	Lightcliffe
Sutton,	Terry	Cleckheaton
Swallow,	Angela	Huddersfield
Tatham,	Andrew and Brenda	Brighouse
Thackray Museum		Leeds
The Hick Family		Scarborough
Thomas,	David and Muriel	Guiseley
Thoresby Society Library		Leeds

List of Subscribers

Tilley,	John and Jean	Colchester
Traynor,	John and Anne	Liversedge
Wade,	John C.	Devon
Walton,	Margaret	Brighouse
Ward,	Derek and Anne	Shibden
Watson,	Wendy and Robert	Hartshead
Wellcome Library		London
Whittingham,	Carole and Francis	Rastrick
Wilkinson,	Ray and Margery	Greetland
Winfield,	Barbara	Guiseley